P9-CAO-548

Patient Practitioner Interaction

An Experiential Manual for Developing the Art of Health Care

ATLANTIC COMM. COLLEGE

Patient Practitioner Interaction

An Experiential Manual for Developing the Art of Health Care

Carol M. Davis, EdD, PT
Graduate Program in Physical Therapy
University of Miami School of Medicine
Coral Gables, FL

SLACK Incorporated, 6900 Grove Road, Thorofare, NJ 08086-9447

dedication

To Jamie

Managing Editor: Amy E. Drummond
Cover Design: Linda Baker
Publisher: John H. Bond

Copyright ©1994 by SLACK Incorporated

All rights reserved. No part of this book may be reproduced, stored in a retrieval system or transmitted in any form or by any means, electronic, mechanical, photocopying, recording or otherwise, without written permission from the publisher, except for brief quotations embodied in critical articles and reviews.

A significant portion of the textual and graphic content of this book was previously published in various forms in another work entitled *Patient Practitioner Interaction: An Experiential Manual For Developing the Art of Health Care, First Edition.*
To order *Patient Practitioner Instructor's Manual* call SLACK Incorporated order department at 1-800-257-8290 or 1-609-848-1000.

Davis, Carol M.
Patient practitioner interaction: an experiential manual for developing the art of health care /   Carol Davis. -- 2nd ed.
   p. cm.
   Includes bibliographical references and index.
   ISBN 1-55642-232-6
   1. Physical therapist and patient. I. Title.
   RM705.D38 1994
   610.69'6--dc20   93-42145
                                  CIP

Printed in the United States of America

Published by: SLACK Incorporated
              6900 Grove Road
              Thorofare, NJ 08086-9447

Last digit is print number: 10   9   8   7   6   5   4   3   2

contents

foreword

An individual's "socialization" into a profession has always been recognized as important, and indeed, inevitable. But only in recent years has the socialization process been viewed as ambipotent, that is, a process carrying the power to effect either positive or negative results for health professionals and society. Thus it is understandable that the idea of socialization is receiving new and careful attention.

Socialization is a joint venture embarked upon by a student, health professionals and society, each adding a unique contribution. Both the content and format of Carol Davis' book invite the student to understand that he/she is an agent in the venture, not an unwitting bystander. The book provides an opportunity for one to engage in and actively reflect upon the socialization process, beginning and ending with the key player, oneself. Correctly it emphasizes that as a student there is a privilege *and* a responsibility to create a role consistent with the health professions' highest ideals.

The health professions' highest ideals have roots in the larger society. The ideals make themselves available to the student; they are instruments whereby a student can prepare to participate *qua* health professional in the protection and fostering of a good society. But the high ideals are not automatically appropriated and fine-tuned by completing a course of professional preparation; the student must confront, reflect upon and choose what type of person he or she wants to be.

Never has a career in the health professions presented a more engaging opportunity for personal enrichment and meaningful societal contribution. Never have so many resources been available to patients who seek to maintain healthy lives or find healing, comfort or rehabilitation. At the same time this embarrassment of riches is held together in a fragile refractory network of competing values and loyalties. Historians tell us that in times of great social upheaval the crystal chalice of a society's most basic values is raised to the sun's rays to see which hues in the spectrum will shine brightest. Our society is in such a period regarding health care, and the causes are multiple. For example, during the second half of the century the introduction of expensive and elaborate medical technology cast a shadow between hands-on clinical approaches of the past and high-technology methods of today. Of what unique value is the human—the health professional—in this interaction with buttons, electrical currents, invisible waves and ah, yes, another human—the patient? Many are asking such questions.

A cartoon in a popular magazine recently portrayed several health professionals, in various postures of consternation, each facing an elaborate apparatus of machines, lights and wires. One is saying, "I give up! Where's the patient?" One can imagine that the patient on the other side of the machinery who is undergoing chemotherapy, a CT scan, an EKG or EMG is asking, "I give up, where's my health professional?" And the health professional may ask additional questions as he or she goes about the day's activities:

"I give up: Why am I here doing all this administrative red tape? I thought I was going to be treating patients!"

"I give up: Where's the professional guideline that has helped health professionals in such situations as I'm in now?"

"I thought the ideals and values would be a clear beacon, but I'm in the dark on this one!"

While technology and other modern influences have raised new questions, there's no need to "give up." The reader of this book will find a light to guide through the shadowy places of new situations. The author systematically, persistently and gracefully raises the chalice of values for the student to examine. The process of examination holds the key to self-understanding, and in the cultivation of self-understanding is the door through which one can walk with confidence into one's career in the health professions.

Ruth Purtilo, P.T., Ph.D.
Boston, Massachusetts

preface
SECOND EDITION

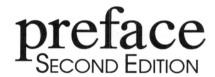

One of the nicest things that happens to you when you write a textbook is that people who know you only from your written work feel free to come up to you in a crowd and begin talking to you about what you've written, as if you were picking up a conversation you'd started long ago. What a pleasure it has been for me to receive feedback from many over the past four years in this and other ways. The nature of my approach has been to use many examples from my life, and so the material in the text really does give readers information with which to converse with me on a more personal basis. I have enjoyed this tremendously, and I thank all of you who have given me helpful suggestions about what worked for you from the first edition, and what didn't.

Chief among the changes in the second edition is the revision of the former Chapter 8, on resolving ethical dilemmas. With the help of detailed and pointed criticism solicited by SLACK, I was encouraged to write a more useful chapter on ethical dilemma resolution which focused on traditional teleological and deontological approaches. By themselves these approaches can be viewed as rather dry, but my pilot research on how clinicians actually go about successfully solving dilemmas helped me to make this chapter more clinically relevant, I believe. A look at the preliminary data from the research revealed the importance of one's moral autobiography which then introduced the use of stories as a way of enhancing one's self awareness regarding the deontological weighing of moral alternatives. The quality of discernment places dilemma resolution in a process that includes both thinking and feeling, the problem solving method which seems to be most successful for professional clinicians. And all of a sudden the material was no longer dry at all! Dilemma resolution with a heart. I expect to hear from the biomedical ethicists.

For help in working through the challenge of improving this part of the book, I am grateful to Harry Benson and Cheryl Willoughby at SLACK for soliciting the reviews of the former Chapter 8. Likewise thank you to the anonymous reviewers who greatly assisted my understanding of how the chapter fell short of doing what I intended it to do. I am most grateful to Herm Triezenberg and Elizabeth Mastrom for introducing the concept of stories to me, and to Elsa Ramsden and Ernie Nalette for helping me expand my thoughts about the nature of resolving dilemmas.

One other substantive improvement to this edition, I believe, comes from my colleague, Kathy Curtis, who helped me to understand the critical importance of attribution theory to assertiveness. In order to use assertiveness skills, you must first believe that something that you say will indeed make a difference. And so this edition of the text encourages the reader to examine one more time the way his or her lenses are set and hopefully assists one to experience a positive outcome for one's self as well as for others.

I've been teaching since 1971, and more than ever I feel grateful for each of my students who helped me to refine this material for maximum usefulness and relevance to them in their professional careers. Every once in awhile I hear from them in serendipitous ways. They share important news with me about their growth and about their professional and personal lives. I feel humble to have walked the path with each of them for awhile, and am grateful when something I teach or have written makes their way easier or more effective.

One of the intentions of this book is to assist the reader in deciding the best thing to do for the patient when the system would insist otherwise. Since the publication of PPI, first edition, my mother died. Her death was an important moment for me in many ways because, along with my twin sister, Susan, I was able to be with her and hold her hand as we kept the 17 hour vigil. We were both tested by a series of events and by people who would have allowed her dying to be more traumatic and painful than it was. Because we persisted in fighting assertively for what we knew she wanted, and what we knew was right and humane to do, she died peacefully and with dignity.

I have come to see that writing this text has helped me to clarify and integrate principles that have resulted in a richer life for me as a health professional. I am grateful for my boss, Sherri Hayes, who encourages me to do the things that I most love to do, I am grateful to my colleagues at the University of Miami and in physical therapy for their collegial support, and for encouraging me to research and write about matters that are not circumscribed by pure thought alone. Most of all I am grateful to my kindred spirits around the world who are ready in a heartbeat to be present to me in all of my incompleteness. They are the ones who assist me with keeping my quadrants balanced. In their hearts, they know who they are, and I am there with them in that knowing. Thank you.

preface
FIRST EDITION

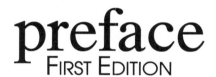

This book is a workbook designed for students and professionals who are willing to embark on a path of growth, specifically, the path of professional socialization. The professional socialization process is an induction into a professional role. When novices become health professionals, they are expected to learn how to act as professionals. Historically it was assumed that this learning how to act would take place automatically along with the incorporation of new knowledge and skill. Students were expected to develop a kind of sixth sense and, with careful observation, grasp the right things to say and do, and discern the right values and attitudes to embody as a professional. If one failed this process of osmosis, he or she stood out from the rest and became suspect.

We now understand the process of professional socialization more adequately, and realize that novices and young professionals can be assisted in learning the professional role. This text is designed to help this process.

How can a text/workbook assist you to grow, to change, to mature, to develop as a mature healing professional? This book represents one aspect of the socialization process that will offer you material to read, reflect upon, respond to, and, in general, experience. The goal is to help you, the reader, to think about various carefully chosen topics in such a way as to raise your consciousness about your "self," about your self interacting with the goal of promoting healing, and about your self working with groups with a professional purpose. Using an interactive format, learning is designed to be personally meaningful and as intense as the reader allows. Hopefully, changes will occur in how well you know yourself, your attitudes will be invited to conform to those believed to promote healing, and your perceptions will become clearer and more global, less idiosyncratic and more in line with the norms and values of healing professions.

The text/workbook format is designed for individual interaction. Part I is devoted to helping you increase awareness of your "self." One's basic attitudes, beliefs and values are rarely examined and less often discussed. But those basic constructs are the framework upon which judgments are made and comprise the fundamental operating principles out of which our perceptions of ourselves and the world emerge. Each of us carries around a kind of voice which tells us things about the world, even when the opinion of that voice isn't asked. What are your basic beliefs about yourself, about people in general, about men versus women, about old people and children, about rapists and murderers? What are your feelings about your body? What perceptions do you have about your communication skills, your ability to be helpful? What right do people have to health care? What is stressful to you? How do you handle stress? What personal values do you consider to be most important? How do those values coincide with the values of compassionate and effective health care?

These beliefs and attitudes lead to a basic philosophy of life which may, in most instances, be quite in harmony with the healing process. But sometimes we find ourselves feeling anxious. Anxiety emerges both when we're not sure what the right thing to do is and when we know the right thing to do, but we don't want to do it. Part I concludes with a chapter that teaches you how to identify and resolve moral or ethical dilemmas.

Part II deals with interaction. The nature of effective helping is explored; a process of assertive therapeutic communication is taught and then expanded to instruction in patient interviewing. A closer look at caring for patients who are dying will assist you in clarifying your ideas about life and death and will give you useful ideas with which to interact in an emotion-laden circumstance. The workbook concludes with a close look at professional stress, or burnout.

These topics represent material I have been using for the last 20 years in my teaching of health professionals. They are offered with the hope that they will assist students and professionals alike in the important growth process on the path to becoming a mature healing professional. Each exercise is followed by an opportunity for you to journal, to write out specific reflections you have about the material just considered. I encourage you to take full opportunity to record your growth as it unfolds.

It is well established that the journaling process is an invaluable aid in the identification of one's feelings as well as one's thoughts. Until you are fully aware of what you feel, as well as think, you unwittingly will act in ways that sometimes don't make sense. A health professional not in full awareness of feelings invites disaster. An invaluable lesson in maturing is to realize that the work that we do will inevitably arouse strong feelings. Feelings happen. We can't block them except at great emotional cost. Alternatively, we can identify them and choose how and when to act on them. And assisting you to know how and when to act appropriately is one of the main goals of this text/workbook.

To assist you in the identification of your feelings, the *Feeling Wheel* (Figure 1) offers a framework that delineates the six basic feelings. The middle circle further refines the basic feelings, and the outer circle describes how one might appear to others while experiencing this emotion. As you journal, if you experience yourself struggling to identify a feeling, this figure might help. College students are overdeveloped in their abilities to intellectualize. Resist the urge to talk about your thoughts and the facts of the situation, and force yourself to journal about what feelings are aroused by the experience. And remember, feelings are one word. "I feel that" is the introduction to a thought, not a feeling. I feel ___ is the expression most useful to discover your emotions around a topic.

This book was first envisioned in Chicago in June of 1986 over lunch with Geneva Johnson, my mentor and friend. Through her encouragement and support I was linked with Harry Benson from SLACK Inc. and the book was conceptualized over lunch in Boston later that year. Harry, Lynn Borders and Cheryl Willoughby at SLACK have been key supporters in this effort, and I thank them for all of their help.

I would like to acknowledge the contributions of all those who have helped me on my path, but the number is great. I would be remiss, however, not to mention the feedback and new learning over the years that I have gleaned from my students, as well as the profound contributions made by Ruth Purtilo, Jane Mathews, Elsa Ramsden, Margaret Moore, Geneva Johnson, Dorothy Pinkston, Don Lehmkuhl, Marjorie Ionta, Dorothy Voss, Marilyn Gossman, Judy Cantey, Brenda Munsey, Helen Hickey, Patricia Yarbrough, Ruth Ouimette, Susan Doughty, Mary Ann Douglas, Victor Kestenbaum, and Jamiss Sebert, not only to my professional life, but to my growth as a person as well. And you see, this is what it is all about. One day you realize that who you are as a person and who you are as a professional have merged, gently, delightfully into a comfortable whole. At that point you feel yourself traveling the road to self actualization. It is my belief that the work you will do with this text will assist you in that vitally important process. So, welcome to a set of experiences designed just for you. Most of all, have fun!

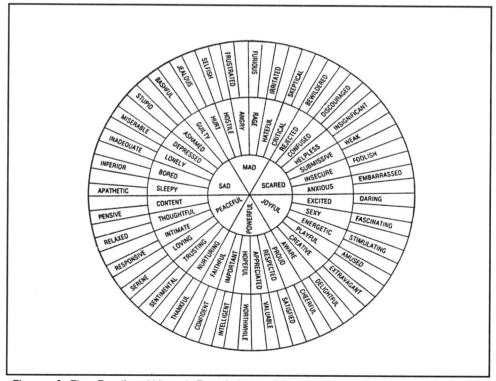

Figure 1. The Feeling Wheel. Reprinted with permission from *Transactional Analysis Journal, Vol 12(4), p. 276.*

section one

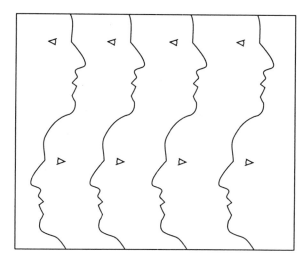

AWARENESS OF SELF

This first section is composed of four chapters: Basic Awareness of Self, Family History, Values as Determinants of Behavior, and Identifying and Resolving Moral Dilemmas. The process of professional maturation requires an in-depth look at who we are at any given time. Who we are includes awareness of our basic ideas, beliefs and feelings about the physical, intellectual, emotional and spiritual aspects of ourselves. These ideas, beliefs and feelings grow out of the sum total of all our experiences, some say even before birth. The first chapter examines some of our basic ideas about ourselves and the perceptions we hold at this particular time of who we are as individuals. The second chapter takes us back to our growing up years and to the memories we have of the influence our family members had on our current beliefs about the world and about ourselves. The third chapter brings us back to the current day, with an invitation to look at our current values, many of which will directly influence the behaviors we manifest in the therapeutic process. The fourth chapter examines how we develop our ideas about right and wrong behavior, based on personal values, and how those values can be compared to the values of a profession.

Each chapter begins with a set of objectives which is designed to point out the goals for learning. In order to really learn about your self and your current values, ideas and communication patterns, it is necessary for you to interact with the content in these pages. Learning implies action, a change in behavior. The more senses involved in the learning process and the more reflection and consideration of thought that the learner expends, the more likely that change will take place in a deep and integrated way. Thus, at the conclusion of each chapter, experiential exercises are offered which are designed to help you achieve the goals for that chapter.

The aim of this book is to teach you how to learn about yourself, about others and about the world in which you interact with others. And so, in essence, this is a beginning for some, and for others a continuation of a lifelong learning that many assert is necessary for effective and compassionate health care. Let's begin!

chapter one

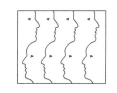

Basic Awareness of Self

Objectives

1. To introduce the concept of the "self."
2. To emphasize the importance of self-knowledge in relation to the quality of one's life and the choices one makes.
3. To facilitate self-awareness through reading, completing exercises and journaling about oneself.

What is the "Self"?

How well do you know yourself? Why would anyone ever ask that question? Some would say that the better you know yourself, the more aware you are of your thoughts and feelings, your strengths and weaknesses, the more you feel in control of your life, then the less stressed and helpless you feel, the less surprised you are by your responses to life. Thus, it might be said that the quality of one's life is, in part, measured by the amount of personal control one feels over day-to-day happenings and choices.

People who are forced to live in institutions to be cared for by others especially feel the negative effect of powerlessness in being forced to succumb to the rules of the larger order, the system. For example, few personal choices are preserved in nursing homes and hospitals.

What is the "self"? How is the self different from the body? What are people asking when they ask, "Who am I, really?" "Why am I here?" These are timeless questions that curiously seem to become more the focus of concern as we live the second half of life than the first. It has been said that the first half of life for many of us is the "doing" half, and the second half of life becomes the "being" half. When we are very busy achieving and working for security and happiness, questions like, "Who am I?" seem distracting. Once we grow beyond our mid 30s, these questions take on greater importance as we reflect on the meaning of life.

Young children are unable to be truly self-aware. But you may remember that delicious moment when you first discovered, all by yourself, that you were uniquely different from anyone in all the world. You were probably six or seven. Richard Zaner, in his text, *The Context of Self*,[1] describes a colleague's recounting of this moment:

> As far as I can tell, I must have been younger than eight years old when I began having what I now call I-am-me experiences. On such occasions I would tell myself insistently, 'This is me, me. . .' (or rather in my native German: 'Das bin ich, ich. . .'). The inner pronouncing of these words and especially the repetition of the personal pronoun were accompanied with the feeling of a cave-in, a dropping down from a surface level of self-awareness to a more and more personal me-myself. Along with it went a feeling of being sucked down as by a whirlpool into a bottomless depth. As I repeated the pronoun 'me' I felt as if one mask after another fell off until the actor behind these masks was stripped to his naked core. (p. 157, 58)

To be able to reflect upon the full nature of "one's self," however, seems to require the cognitive skills and experience of a person with a mature nervous system. To become aware of oneself, one must go outside of oneself and ponder the self and, for example, analyze one's motives for behavior. This only becomes possible, according to Piaget, at the stage of formal operations.[2]

The Desire for Self-Awareness

The wish to become self-aware often has to do with the search for meaning in life and the desire to experience a choice in the process of who one is becoming. In other words, the question, "Who am I?" is necessary before one can truly be who one chooses to be.

Parents tell children how to act most often with good intention. Most children are socialized into becoming what their parents or guardians believe are good human beings who will live happy and productive lives. The influence of the family on one's self-esteem and self-concept is a very important topic that will be covered in more depth in Chapter Two.

The goal of health professional education is to assist students in becoming a certain way: professional. What does it mean to "be professional"? Much has been written elsewhere about that question. Suffice it to say here that any description of a professional would contain the integration of a body of knowledge and skills and the proficient and effective delivery of the same. In the profession of health care, proficient and effective delivery requires, I believe, a "therapeutic use of one's self" while interacting with clients. Superior skill in the technology of the profession must be balanced with the art of relating to those who request our services in such a way that healing is facilitated rather than interfered with.

If health care consisted of "working on bodies" alone, perhaps a consideration of the self would not be necessary. But the fact remains that health care involves people interacting with people in such a way that what is not right is correctly analyzed and appropriately influenced so that it is changed to approximate more closely what is right. This analysis and influence takes place between human beings who have not just brought their bodies to us, but have brought their feelings, their fears, their hopes, their frustrations, their pain. Illness is meaningful only as it is lived, moment to moment. When we care professionally, we care for people living their illness, not for broken bodies.

Let's take a closer look at the nature of the "self," what it is, what it is not, how it grows and is influenced, and how it performs as we mature into healthy, more "self-actualized" human beings.

The Self

Human beings are tremendously complex organisms, capable of portraying various identities or roles depending on what the situation calls for or stimulates. Much study has been devoted to the manner in which we can divide ourselves into various parts or take on different roles and yet still remain essentially the same person, or "whole." Transactional analysis literature teaches about the "parent, adult and child" in each of us.[3] We each portray various roles throughout the day, such as employee, boss, sister, brother, friend. Carl Jung, in his attempt to explore the nature of the unconscious, described archetypal elements present in all personalities. Among them were the persona, the shadow and the self.[4] Freud is famous for his explications of the ego, the id and the superego. All of these now rather common terms were created to help explain the complex behavior of human beings.

The psychology literature informs us about the nature of the self and its role in human growth by way of Figure 1-1.

This figure represents the various layers of a person, or the various aspects of a personality. The outermost layer is best described as the persona, or the public face each of us puts on in the world in order to appear in control, intelligent, witty, sensitive and lovable.[4] We act in the ways we believe are going to bring us love and recognition. But deep inside we know that the persona is really a mask. Underneath that mask is another aspect of

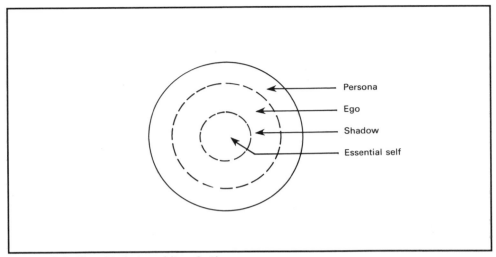

Figure 1-1. The Nature of the Self.

ourselves that is filled with doubts and insecurities. Almost all of us are dissatisfied with living our lives totally from behind the mask. Each of us desires to drop our false fronts and to become who we truly are, to express ourselves more honestly, to be more truly ourselves and to be loved for it.[5]

The second layer can be seen to be composed of the ego, or the center of the conscious mind as described by Freud, and the shadow, the unconscious, "natural" side of our personalities.[4] The ego is the part of us that gets the job of living done. It is the force that gets us through school, that makes choices for us that are designed, as best we can know, to bring us happiness. It problem solves for us and helps us have the courage to act and the patience to wait. But the ego is made up of all kinds of misinformation about ourselves and about the world. Egos tend to be very protective; they tend to move us toward safety, toward the status quo. The ego believes in its own omnipotence. But it has to sustain that belief by using a lot of energy, and by ignoring many messages that would refute that omnipotence. The feeling of godlikeness of the ego is an illusion. In fact, the ego is filled with erroneous ideas and fears about the world and about ourselves. Our egos tell us we're very intelligent one minute, and the next they tell us we're totally naive and stupid. One minute they tell us the world is a wonderful, loving place and the next that it's a dangerous place.

Each of us tends to listen to the still, small voice of the ego when we have to make important choices, but we become very confused about what is important and true. That's because we tend to allow the voice of the ego to reflect what we've heard from important people in our lives about ourselves. If we heard, "You are so stupid, you'll never amount to anything" when we were young, we believed that for a time, until we had the power to prove that it wasn't true. As we achieved success, we told our egos, "See, I really am bright. I *can* succeed!" But instead of dropping the old data and incorporating the new, the ego holds onto the whole package, and spits both messages at us at times when we feel most unable to modify that quiet voice.

The shadow is the unconscious part of this second layer. It is our inferior side, the part of us that wants to do all the things our ego tells us we can't do.[7] When we say things like, "I wasn't myself," or "I don't know what came over me," we're acknowledging the presence of our unconscious shadow that tricks us into behaving in ways we say we abhor.

Underneath these outer two layers, at the center of the person, lies the rest of us, the "more" that the outer two layers can't fully incorporate: the "self." The self is the essence of the person, and incorporates both conscious and unconscious elements of the person into itself.[4] I have my persona, I have my ego, I have my personality, I have my body, I have my possessions in life. . .I *am* my self. The self is the irreducible energy of my uniqueness. It is the thing that makes me absolutely unique in all the world, in spite of the fact that, for example, I have an identical twin sister, and probably thousands of people share my name. It is that marvelous essence of me that I approach as the masks are, one by one, stripped away in the search for what is undividable, what is at my core. It is the unfolding answer to the eternal question, "Who am I, really?"

The self is that energy that can linger for days before the moment of the "crossing over" into death of the physical body. Those who care for the terminally ill have often experienced the phenomenon that, for a time before the body stops functioning totally, it is more accurate to say that all that remains in the bed is a shell that looks like the person's body. The essence of the person seems to "come and go," little by little spending more time gone than present.[5]

The self has to do with the energy inside each human that reincarnationists say is a piece of the deity that is never created or destroyed. It is my "higher self." Christians would call it the "Christ self" within each of us. It exists for all time; it always has and it always will. And the task of human beings on earth is to house this energy as we grow and change, lifetime after lifetime, with the end goal of becoming more like God, like truth.

Jung[4] says this about the nature of the self:

> The self. . .can include both the conscious and the unconscious. It appears to act as something like a magnet to the disparate elements of the personality and the processes of the unconscious, and is the centre of this totality as the ego is the centre of consciousness, for it is the function which unites all the opposing elements in man and woman, consciousness and unconsciousness, good and bad, male and female, etc., and in so doing transmutes them. To reach it necessitates acceptance of what is inferior in one's nature, as well as what is irrational and chaotic. This state cannot be reached by a mature person without considerable struggle; it implies suffering, for the Western mind, unlike the Eastern, does not easily tolerate paradoxes. [The self] consists. . .in the awareness on the one hand of our unique natures, and on the other of our intimate relationship with all life, not only

human, but animal and plant, and even that of inorganic matter and the cosmos itself. It brings a feeling of 'oneness,' and/or reconciliation with life, which now can be accepted as it is, not as it should be. (p. 63)

Thus, the self, once uncovered, seems to hold the real truth about us as human beings. It is our connection with the Truth, and it is out of this center of our existence that we come to feel at-oneness with our fellow human beings. It is the self that is able to cross over in empathy and experience and feel what a moment in life must be like for another person. It is the self that we return to as we quiet our working minds in meditation.

It is the self that allays our fears, that gives us true courage rather than braggadocio or false bravado; it is the self that feels the essential goodness of our humanness, in the face of our incompleteness; it is the self that grows in wisdom and becomes more as we mature, approaching the all-knowing goodness of Truth; it is the self that enables us to laugh at our egos and forgive the well-meaning unkindnesses visited upon us by parents and relatives as they tried desperately to get us to "act right" as children and thereby systematically helped to destroy our inborn connectedness with our true selves.

Self-Awareness

Carl Rogers has said, "It appears that the goal the individual most wishes to achieve, the end which he knowingly and unknowingly pursues, is to become himself."[6] How do we become our selves? How do we discover our true natures? How do we access the self? How do we get close to it, get right up next to it? It begins when we recognize the burning desire to be known for who we are, not for who we believe others want us to be. It begins when we are willing to shed the roles we've assumed in order to win attention and affection and acceptance, and instead commit to being truthful and honest. Often the first steps we take in this direction come with our challenges to our parents and the "rules of the house."

Self-awareness requires reflection in order to ascertain who we truly are. The ego will work overtime to tell you about yourself, but it takes time and an effort of a different sort to reflect deeper, to the messages of the true self.

Often we need help in this process, for our perceptions are unavoidably colored by the messages we heard when we were very young. To sift through unchallenged truths that were reinforced for years (for instance, all women are emotional, all men are insensitive) requires, for example, the perspectives of literature, art, and music and the professional preparation of counselors and psychologists to help us examine our habitual assumptions. The goal of growth of this sort is to expand the narrow, parochial views we held as children, and become more aware of a wider world view that incorporates diversity, that trades black and white, dualistic thinking for the wonderful colors of ambiguity, free from the need to be "right," free from the fear of being "wrong." It is, in a sense, the search for truth that we're after as we mature in our world view. We want to enfold all possibilities rather than leave out information that might be critical for comprehending the complexities of ourselves, of our lives, of the world we live in. In the search for the self the goal becomes to give up beliefs that entrap us in negativity and doubt, and replace them with beliefs that enlarge our consciousness and help us feel compassion for our oneness with all of life.

Search for the Self

This text is designed to help you examine your values, your beliefs, your communication patterns in an effort to assist you in the search for *your* self and to broaden your world view. For it is from the self that we give health care of the highest quality. It is the self that has the capacity to see clearly, to display compassion in the face of threat or fatigue, that "crosses over" in empathy. It is the self that sets appropriate boundaries and refuses to attempt to have personal needs met by patients. It is the self that has unlimited patience and great understanding. It is the self that comprehends the need to be ethical and act with integrity. It is the self that has the desire and the capability to feel unconditional positive regard, and a oneness with all living beings that cancels out judgment and prejudice.

It is the frightened ego, however, that pities and pretends that it is displaying compassion; it is the frightened ego that defends itself rather than offering a healing response to the angry patient; it is the ego that needs to be puffed up and made to feel important at the expense of others' feelings. It is the frightened ego that requires our patients to do as we say, to get better, to thank us for helping them.

All of us want essentially the same thing: to be respected, to be treated with unconditional positive regard. But all of us want that positive acceptance of our whole being, not just of our persona, not just of our ego. We want others to love and accept us as we are wholly, in all of our incompleteness.

The more the ego tries to defend itself, the more difficult it is to catch a glimpse of our selves, our essential natures. If you have been told that you tend to respond defensively to people, you developed this coping skill out of necessity. But it is not very useful in patient care. This will be a good opportunity for you to examine the messages you're receiving that make you feel as if you must defend yourself. Defensiveness always obliterates the truth. It is noisy and useless; it has no sense of humor at all. It is the mark of a person responding to life from an insecure ego, not the sign of a whole and integrated self that might respond to criticism, for example, with, "I didn't know I was coming across that way. I'll take a closer look at my behavior now."

Signs of Growth in Self-Awareness

As people struggle to become more themselves, usually out of the painful realization that the masks they've been using are no longer bringing them happiness and love, Rogers[6] describes them as changing in noticeable ways. They seem to:

1. Drop the defensive mask with which they have faced life, and begin to discover and to experience the stranger who lives behind these masks—the hidden part of self.
2. Emerge with a tendency to be more open to all elements of experience; growing in trust in one's organism as an instrument of sensitive living.
3. Accept the responsibility of being a unique person.
4. Develop the sense of living in life as a participant in a fluid, ongoing process, continually discovering new aspects of one's self in the flow of experience. (p. 124)

When we live daily with an awareness of our true selves, negative feelings are confronted and the beliefs behind them are analyzed and replaced with beliefs that are more positive and cosmic. Thus we take responsibility for creating our own reality, moment to moment. No longer do we allow ourselves to get away with such beliefs as, "You make me so angry." We acknowledge that we make ourselves angry in response to someone, because of a belief we have about that person or that behavior. And then we search for a larger, more hopeful and understanding belief that will replace feelings of negativity.

Conclusion

The goal of this entire text is to assist you in learning more about your self, so that the way in which you relate to patients who come to you for help might be sensitive, compassionate and free from prejudice and negativity. Central to this goal is the assumption that our true or essential selves reflect the essential goodness in all of us, and can be covered up by the persona, the many masks we wear and by the ego that sees the world through lenses that were originally set when we were very young and helpless. The behaviors that facilitate healing as we apply our technology are those behaviors and those underlying beliefs that bring about wholeness and oneness. Behaviors that interfere with healing result in fragmentation, discord, negativity. I believe that it is possible to grow such that the nature of our essential selves is accessible to us, and that, out of a connectedness with our essential selves, we are empowered to provide health care of the highest order. In that connectedness with our essential selves, we have the power to realize the fears and shortcomings of our egos, the falseness and manipulation of our personas. And out of that connectedness with our essential selves we can be the persons we were created to be—capable of unconditional positive regard for all humans. This is the greatest calling of the health care professional. It is a tremendously challenging task to grow to this goal. But the rewards are indescribable.

References

1. Zaner, R: *The Context of Self.* Athens, Ohio, Ohio University Press, 1981.
2. Piaget, J: *The Construction of Reality in the Child.* New York, Basic Books, 1954.
3. Berne, E: *Transactional Analysis in Psychotherapy.* New York, Grove Press, 1961.
4. Fordham, F: *An Introduction to Jung's Psychology.* Baltimore, Penguin Books, 1953.
5. Challoner, HK: *The Wheel of Rebirth.* Wheaton, Ill., The Theosophical Publishing House, 1969.
6. Rogers, C: *On Becoming a Person.* Boston, Houghton Mifflin, 1961.

exercises

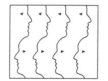

1. What's So About Me?

On a separate sheet of paper that you can keep confidential, answer each of the following as honestly as you can for this moment. Allow at least half a sheet of paper for each question. Each question requires reflection, but jot down the first thing that comes to mind, then take time with each question to clearly communicate your awareness (or lack of it)! You may wish to complete the entire set over a period of a week or so, taking one or two questions at a time.

What's So About Me

Date:

1. I would describe myself as. . .
2. Others would describe me as. . .
3. I am proudest of. . .
4. I was most embarrassed when I. . .
5. I am most annoyed about myself when I. . .
6. I get angriest when. . .
7. Under severe stress I usually. . .
8. Aspects of my communication that I want to keep and refine are. . .
9. Aspects of my communication that I want to change include. . .
10. What I want others to understand about me is that. . .
11. I'm most anxious that. . .
12. Characteristics of other people that impress me most include. . .
13. I protect myself when. . .
14. I would be willing to die in six months if. . .
15. I don't know how to say. . .
16. People are essentially (good, bad, neutral)?. . .
17. Goals I want to achieve

    a. With this course. . .

    b. In my lifetime. . .

Discussion

Once you've answered these questions, write a description about yourself from what you've discovered. Are you totally happy with yourself at this point? What would you change? What did you learn about yourself that will assist you in being a health professional? What may detract from your effectiveness? How aware are you of the messages from your ego, of your shadow? How aware are you of your self? Identify responses that have a negative aspect to them. What is the belief that you hold, that makes that answer true for you? What is an alternative belief that you also hold that would replace the negative one so that your response might be more positive and hopeful?

Example: I protect myself when I am criticized for being too unscientific, too naive or idealistic. Negative belief: I lack the intellect to scientifically prove what I believe is true and important. Replacement belief: The scientific method holds one way of verifying what is true. The balance of logic and facts with intuitive knowing together frames a larger truth. I have proven skills as a scientist and I have faith in my intuition. Both serve me well in my work.

2. Authenticity/Autonomy Self Assessment Tool

At this moment:

1. How in control of your life do you feel?

| 0 | 1 | 2 | 3 | 4 | 5 | 6 | 7 |

Totally helpless
A victim

Total control
over my life

2. How in control do you expect to feel?

1½ years from now (graduation)

| 0 | 1 | 2 | 3 | 4 | 5 | 6 | 7 |

2½ years from now

| 0 | 1 | 2 | 3 | 4 | 5 | 6 | 7 |

5 years from now

| 0 | 1 | 2 | 3 | 4 | 5 | 6 | 7 |

3. How well do you know yourself—who you *really* are and who you really are meant to be, unique in all the world?

| 0 | 1 | 2 | 3 | 4 | 5 | 6 | 7 |

Not a clue;
I constantly
surprise myself

Very familiar
with who I am
and am becoming

4. How well do you accept yourself as you are?

| 0 | 1 | 2 | 3 | 4 | 5 | 6 | 7 |

Dislike myself
very much;
difficult to
accept any part
of me

Very comfortable
with who I am,
how I am in the
world

5. What are some goals you have in order to obtain the "good life," a life that's good for you?

1.

2.

3.

4.

5.

C Davis 2/87

Reflections from this exercise:

3. Collage

With the use of any material, construct a collage that represents you as you know yourself at this moment. Your collage may be comprised of pictures and colors as is the traditional collage, or you may wish to use other materials to construct a less traditional "montage." Do not choose representations of your persona only. Search your heart for symbols of your true self, the part of you that you hold dear but that you do not readily reveal. Also, choose representatives of your ego and your shadow as well. Bring your creation to class wrapped so others cannot identify it. Gather in small groups, place one creation in the center of the group and observe it carefully, *without speaking* for two or three minutes. Gather a private impression of what the creator was trying to convey. Then, in turn, offer observations that you perceive about the person for five minutes or so. After this anonymous discussion, identify the creator. He or she then responds to what was observed by classmates, what was "on target" and where classmates missed the mark. Finally, group members should share what each learned about this classmate before bringing forth the next creation.

Journal

At the conclusion of these exercises, begin a journal about yourself at this time. Journal entries are most useful in learning about yourself if they relate what you learned from the experience. Most of us confuse the concept of a journal with a diary. A diary is designed to record significant events in one's life. A journal is a letter to yourself, designed to stimulate reflection about an experience, rather than just recording the experience. One way to keep from simply recording the event is to begin each entry with the following phrases.

What I felt during the exercise.

What I learned about myself.

So what? Significance or meaning of my learning.

Your journal should be kept in a book with a cover, on pages that do not easily become dislodged. Entries are to be written, ideally, following each exercise, but at the minimum following each chapter. Many find it useful to journal as a way of privately discussing the chapter and its personal significance, as well. Your journal is what you make it. Most university students are unaccustomed to this sort of activity, however, and some abhor writing. For a short time, make a commitment to this activity. Don't forget to use the "Feeling Wheel" which precedes Chapter One. Remember, this journal is by you, for your personal use. Set aside the time on your calendar and once you get into it, I suspect it will become rewarding. Your course instructor may wish to see your entries now and again to be sure you are keeping up. In that case, confidentiality may become more limited. *You will not be graded on your journal.* Since it is a collection of your feelings and reflections, a grade would be wholly inappropriate. However, the value of the activity is such that your instructor may collect it to check your discipline with the activity, and may comment on how well you reflected on the experience rather than simply describing what happened.

chapter two

FAMILY HISTORY

Objectives

1. To describe, in general terms, the role families play in the formation of identity and self esteem.
2. To examine the development of a mature personality as described by Erikson.
3. To introduce the concept of the "false self" in relation to the "true self" as it develops in dysfunctional families.
4. To stress the importance of self-awareness to authenticity or the awareness of the "true self" as opposed to the "false self," and to stress the importance of authenticity to effective, mature helping.

It has been said that a clinician's most important tool is the effective use of self. Our personalities and our styles of relating have everything to do with how effective we are in facilitating the healing process. No one wants to be treated unkindly, least of all when we're not feeling well. Yet unkindness abounds in health care settings. If we would ask health professionals to assess their ability to relate effectively with people, few would admit to lapses in temper, prejudicial behavior, irritability or cutting sarcasm. Yet these and other negative behaviors occur with great frequency.

More difficult to observe are such negative behaviors as lack of honesty, breaking confidences, lack of fidelity to one's colleagues and causing a patient to become overly dependent on oneself.

You might ask, "Why be a health professional if you can't act in ways that are positive and assist healing?" Often clinicians are unaware of their behavior or its effect on others. Patients challenge our sensitivity and maturity in unique ways. Patients react out of the stress of their illness or pain, but practitioners, also, must work under stress, the stresses unique to health care. It requires great maturity and patience to respond in healing ways in less than ideal situations.

Influence of the Family on Self Esteem

Each of us views the world from a unique perspective. I like to use the analogy of a pair of lenses to illustrate one's world view. You and I can be looking at the exact same thing, but what I see and hear and feel and experience generally will be different from what you experience because my "lenses" are set differently from yours. We receive our lenses as small children. One's world view evolves out of what one hears and experiences as a child growing up in a unique family unit. Indeed, we actually develop in the ways that our parents would have us develop because we are, to them, an image on their lenses. Even twins, growing up under the same circumstances, will develop differences in their lenses, based on what each chooses to attend to, to ponder, to emphasize.

Children are not little adults, as Piaget first clearly described.[1] Children have under-developed nervous systems, and lack the capacity to move, think and act in the ways that adults can. Children live in a land of make-believe, enjoy fantasy and are egocentric. They are unable to handle abstract logic, and are very present oriented and concrete. If you ask a child which of two parallel, identical pencils is longer, she'll say, correctly, that both are the same length. But then if you slide one pencil so that it is ahead of the other, though still parallel, and then ask, "Which pencil is longer?" she'll say the pencil that is ahead of the other is longer. In other words, children can't conserve information. Likewise, children are unable to come outside of themselves and view themselves, as we discussed in Chapter One. Ask a child who has a brother if he has a brother and he'll say, "Yes." Ask him if his brother has a brother, he'll say, "No."[2]

Finally, children idolize their parents. Feelings of helplessness and dependence are coped with by believing that Mommy and Daddy are perfect and no harm can come to me as long as they are with me in life.

Erik Erikson[3] has developed a useful description of the development of personality (Table 2-1) that centers on the successful resolution of tension in a series of dialectical steps encountered by the growing person from birth onward. A certain degree of accomplishment is required with each stage as it is encountered, or the child will have to master the goal later. This is similar to the child who skips crawling, wherein critical movements necessary to accomplished gait remain absent. There is a certain level of suffering or pathology that results, even if one seems to be functioning adequately. Table 2-1 summarizes Erikson's theory of development. We will return to this theory in Section Two when we discuss the development of effective helping behaviors.

Human beings are among the few living creatures born without the capacity to crawl, wiggle or walk to a source of food. It might be said that we are nine months in the womb and nine (or more) months out, totally helpless to move about to a source of food or nourishment.

Table 2-1.
Psychosocial Theory of Development: A Summary of Erikson's Epigenetic Stages of Development

Trust vs. Mistrust (0-12 months)

From birth to approximately one year, this stage is the basis for all future development of personality. A feeling of physical comfort accompanied by minimal fear and uncertainty results in a sense of trust for the infant. The quality of the relationship with mother or maternal figure is more important than quantity of food or love demonstrations. Experiences with one's body are the first and primary means of social interactions for the baby, thus they provide the foundations for psychological trust. The issues involved in trust and mistrust are not settled for all time during this phase of life; they may arise again and again during development and later life. Later confrontation with trust may shake one's basic trust, or provide another opportunity for further development if these needs were not met adequately the first time.

Autonomy vs. Shame and Doubt (2-4 years)

As the child of two to four experiences the world around him, he begins to discover that his behavior can bring about certain results. Out of these encounters with reality grows a sense of autonomy. At the same time the child has some conflicts about asserting or remaining dependent and in which situations. Exploring is a primary goal of this growing and increasingly coordinated physical being. It becomes more and more difficult to remain in a confined place. The child is occupied with activities involving retaining and releasing—manipulating objects, expressing himself, making new friends and letting them go, and bodily functions. The degree to which the child will allow others to regulate his behavior is regularly tested, leading to a greater sense of self understanding and responsibility. Or in the case of over control, leading to shame and doubt.

Initiative vs. Guilt (4-5 years)

During the fourth and fifth years, language development and locomotion have reached a sufficiently high level to permit expansion of imagination. Play activities are more interesting and companionship with peers is sought. There is curiosity and comparison with others around size and skill issues; who is the better tree climber, who is biggest or best at—almost anything. The child in this stage is into everything and seeks attention verbally and physically. Sexual curiosity and genital stimulation are apparent. Adult treatment of the curiosity will reinforce the initiative or result in shame and guilt. Because of a very active imagination, the child may feel guilty for the mere thoughts, and for activities which no one has observed. The evolving conscience is becoming established and will ultimately control initiative. If the child's activities are perceived as a nuisance, whether motor or verbal, it may develop feelings of guilt over self-initiated activities which may last a lifetime. Healthy identification with parents, teachers, and peers help resolve some of the guilt problems.

Industry vs. Inferiority (6-11 years)

Between the ages of 6 and 11 the child moves seriously into the world of competition, and the separation of work and play. The individuals having impact on the developing sense of self now include many other adults and a wider sphere of peers. As the lessons of work are learned, the child often needs to slip into the familial play world to bolster what may feel like flagging initiative. The developing industry evolves from efforts and achievement rewarded by significant others and leads to a sense of social worth. When the child learns social worth is linked to background of parents, color of skin, or the label on his clothes, identity with those conditions rather than self may result. These first four stages form the base upon which the adolescent builds a sense of identity.

Identity vs. Identity Diffusion (12-18 years)

During this stage of changes, the consistent task is striving to be oneself and to share oneself with something else. The beginning of separation from parents finally becomes a serious agenda. The adolescent experiences the need to be master of his own affairs and to be free of dependency. The emerging young adult is eager to know his abilities and to have the adult world recognize them as well. The adolescent also fears that the demands of adulthood will exceed the capacities to

---

Table 2-1 continued.

meet them. Time perspective versus time diffusion becomes the dilemma. When the adult world offers the adolescent responsibilities and privileges at an appropriate pace, commensurate with capacity and desires, there is resolution of some of the issues with a sense of time perspective, as opposed to urgency and hopelessness. The derivatives of the second stage of "autonomy versus shame and doubt" are reworked in the adolescent in the form of establishing a sense of self certainty. When adult(s) can offer reinforcement appropriately to build the adolescent's self esteem, feelings of inferiority diminish. The remains of "initiative versus guilt" reappear with the need to discover individualized and unique talents and interest. There seems to be a need to experiment with different roles and express initiative in different ways. If stymied in this dimension, it may seem easier to resolve the conflict by seeking behavior or roles in conflict with parents or the community—thus achieving a negative identity which is preferable to an "identity diffusion" which is experienced as being nobody at all. Most authorities agree that the period of adolescence brings with it an increase in psychic energy. The young person who uses these energies effectively can experiment in many ways and have experiences of achievement. If much of the energy is used to resolve feelings resulting from earlier unresolved crises, which often reappear at this time, then the rather fragile sense of self may be seriously threatened, with introspection interfering with concentration. The successful resolution of adolescent tasks and the development of a strong sense of identity may require many years beyond age 18. During this time the young adult experiments with new behavior and may ignore some societal mores in the process. It is important for this process to work itself through, especially with talented and creative persons. Negative labeling may reinforce a temporary identity which, given time, will work itself into something else.

Intimacy vs. Isolation

The first phase of adulthood comes into being after the adolescent has worked out a sense of identity. Sexual and psychological intimacies between two people while retaining one's own identity is the primary task of this stage. This goal is sought through forms of friendship, leadership, athletics, even combat. Unwillingness or inability to achieve intimacy will result in distancing oneself from others who pose a threat to identity. Achievement is characterized by the ability and willingness to share with another in mutual trust, to regulate cycles of work, and to participate in society in self satisfying ways. This stage continues through early middle age.

Generativity vs. Stagnation

The basic agenda of the middle years is aimed at guiding the next generation, whether in parenting or through employment and enjoyment situations. The critical question of this time occurs when the individual looks back to examine what has happened up to that time in life and whether it was good. If the individual turns inward and becomes self-absorbed, stagnation results.

Integrity vs. Despair

The primary task of the later years is the acceptance of one's self and one's life. When the individual has experienced the feelings that accompany a share of the good things of life without being overwhelmed by its tragedies, disappointments and frustrations, ego integrity is the result. There is acceptance of one's existence with full responsibility and commitment to a certain way of life and its values. Having experienced what is felt to be a full life, the individual can accept giving it up with "integrity." If on the other hand the person feels there has been little good from life and there are few prospects of any coming, there is a sense of despair often accompanied by fear of death.

Reprinted with permission from Ramsden E: Affective dimensions in patient care. In Payton O. (ed): *Psychosocial Aspects of Clinical Practice*. NY, Churchill Livingstone, 1986.

We lie there, like blobs, and must wail and cajole to get the attention of the big people around us in order to get our basic survival needs met.

The fact that we are born totally dependent on others for our survival is a critical aspect of the development of our world view, for who we are and how the world is for us depends totally on how we are responded to in our profound neediness, and on what we hear others say to us and about us. As a child, I have no identity save what others say about me. It is obvious that the maturity of the parent, and the extent to which the child is wanted and anticipated have a great deal to do with how the parent responds to the child, and thus fosters or inhibits the development of a sense of self-identity, and self-esteem.

Few of us grew up in ideal homes. Perhaps you think you are the exception. The fact is that we experience denial, and many of us have difficulty remembering the negative things about our childhoods. Remember that little children all think that their parents are perfect. Adolescents give up those notions, but replace them with strongly held mores to honor parents and respect them. If parents were emotionally or physically abusive to a child, the child will automatically believe it was her fault, for she must have been bad. Part of maturation is to give up our idealized views of our parents. No parents are perfect. Ironically, however, the more abandoned the child was, the more she clings to the fantasy of how perfect her parents were. To idealize your parents is to idealize the way they raised you.[2] It is very important to look back at what was happening in your family when you were growing up as one mechanism to increase your awareness of your self and your world view. What do you remember about the circumstances of your birth? Were you a wanted child?

Each child is born into a unique and complex family situation and encounters various challenges, as described by Erikson, as he or she develops day by day. If I, as a newborn, experience feelings of physical comfort, emotional calm and joy at my presence, if my needs are attended to with love and compassion, I will develop a sense of trust and the view that the world is essentially a warm and loving place. If, for example, something happens to my mother, however, and I become a burden to others left to care for me, and people are mourning the loss of my mother and harbor resentment toward me for causing her loss, I will experience a different set of feelings, and may believe that the world is uncertain and chaotic in nature. If I am born to a 15-year-old who needs love and attention still from her parents, who has little love to give and should be giving it to herself, the situation becomes cruelly different. Very likely she can't stand to hear me cry and may beat and smother me when I do. If that is the case, I will experience the world as a hostile place, and I will mistrust from the very first days of my life. This scenario is the genesis of violent adolescents out of control, so prevalent in our contemporary society.

And so we develop inwardly; we set our emotional lenses in response to the way our maturing nervous system takes in the information around us. At about age two we are confronted with the need to be toilet trained. This is reflected in Erikson's second stage, Autonomy versus Shame and Doubt (Table 2-1). Some children are placed on the "potty" at six months, before head control occurs, let alone complete myelinization of the nerves. As the description on the table suggests, a critical learning at this stage is the child's appropriate and balanced willingness to allow others to regulate and control his or her behavior. Autonomy results in the feeling of success free from shame and guilt. Shame and guilt result when the child is unable to succeed and consequently allows the adult to over control his or her behavior. Only shame, or the feeling that, "I am bad" can result when a child is placed on a potty and told to urinate when she doesn't even know what that means or how it feels to control that function because she cannot yet feel sensation in those nerves. However, when the child is fully ready for this learning, a marvelous feeling of success and pride results with being able to "make bubbles" in the water on command.

It is unrealistic to believe that each stage of development might be totally successfully conquered. Children will have successful resolution at times, and will suffer unsuccessful resolution at times. The point that I want to stress is that the balance toward more successful resolution than unsuccessful has a great deal to do with parents and other adults who don't set children up to fail. Parents who do not parent well were, themselves, not parented well. Dysfunctional parents learned to be dysfunctional from the families they grew up in.

Current self-awareness is assisted by an attempt to remember (and to ask the help of others who watched one grow through) critical stages in development over the years. How we respond to the world today is greatly influenced by our sense of ourself and the adequacy of our self-esteem. The development of a healthy self-esteem requires more successful than unsuccessful resolution of the tensions described by Erikson either as we mature, or later. As adults we can examine our growing up experiences, gain insight into our dysfunctional views and consciously change our distorted world view, or correct our lenses, to give us a more true and accurate focus of the world and of ourselves. However, we usually enter into this examination only because we're experiencing emotional pain or we're bored with our lives.

Healthy or Open Families

Healthy families interact in ways that have been described as "open" in contrast to the rigid or "closed" functioning of troubled or dysfunctional families (Table 2-2). A family functions to provide a safe and supportive environment for all of its members to learn basic values, to grow and become more fully human. In healthy families, members feel empowered to adapt to change and feel supported in coping with the stresses of the world both outside the home and within. The stress inside the home is usually perceived to be less than the stress faced outside in the world, except in transient phases of family crisis. Individuals are recognized as being unique and having worth. There is value to the family unit, and there is open communication where members feel free to speak their opinion, but do so with concern and caring for others. In sum, family members feel safe, supported, encouraged and appreciated.

Table 2-2. Characteristics of Families		
Open/Healthy	**Troubled**	**Closed/Unhealthy**
Open to change Flexible responses to each situation	Nothing can be done What's the use?	Rigid, fixed, harsh rules Right vs. wrong, no exceptions
High self worth People are valued as individuals	Shaky self worth Cover feelings of low self control	Evasive responses Low self worth, lots of shaming behavior Low ownership—blaming
Functional defenses Uses defenses as coping skill with insight	Use defenses to hide pain Defenses more often deny real feelings *Choice is lost* Always smile or cry or complain, etc.	*No Choice*—react compulsively & rigidly out of fear. Short fuses. Lots of avoidance or rage.
Clear rules discussed Hours, respect for property, telephone use, chores, etc. regularly negotiated.	Unclear—rules inconsistent Depends on who is asked what day, which child, etc.	Edicts or no rules at all Chaos—rules cannot be followed
People take risks to express feelings, ideas, beliefs	Not safe to express feelings or give opinions. "Don't rock the boat." Can't disagree.	Denial of problems Ignore bizarre behaviors No talk rule—even about serious problems, especially drinking, drugs.
Can deal with stress, pick up on other's pain. Nurturing & caring for each other. Seek out those in pain to support, encourage.	Avoid pain Do not see it in others. Sweep problems under the rug. Pretend all is okay.	Denial of stress Can't cope with any more—glazed eyes don't see pain. Ignore basic need to be seen, acknowledged. Children become early helpers.
Accepts life stages, welcomes them. Celebrate growth—sexuality, new friends, accomplishments	Parents may compete with kids—growth is accepted painfully—don't talk about sex Try to keep children dependent	Passage of time is ignored—change is feared—adults treated as children—children may try to act like adults. Children ridiculed, teased but try to become helpful.
Either clear hierarchy or egalitarian—strong parental coalition—less need to control—can negotiate	*Hidden coalitions* across generations—parental coalition weak—rigid or shifting pattern of domination	Either upside down family—children may run it, or chaotic—no giving out of rules, or one parent in charge of all and can't cope.
Affect is open Direct expression of feelings—all feelings are okay—anger is in context of awareness of other person. Considerate of others	Negativism, low feeling, bickering, argumentative controlled mood, some feelings okay, some not, inconsistent acceptance of feelings	Cynicism, open hostility, violence, sadism—actually try to manipulate & hurt each other. Only happiness is allowed.

Roles and responsibilities of members are flexible but clear. People function well day to day and in crisis. Finally, quality time is shared by parents and children and is enjoyed.

Sadly few of us grew up in ideal situations, and very few of us received all that we needed to mature as healthy, fully functioning, mature true selves.

Dysfunctional or Closed Families

Charles Whitfield believes that many people grow up in families that stifle the development of the true self and instead cultivate in the child a false or "co-dependent" self.[5] Children need to feel as if they are safe and protected at all times. They need to feel free to ask questions, to run and play, to know that the boundaries that parents set for them are fair and consistent. Children need to feel as if they can be children, learning and growing without fear of being ridiculed or punished cruelly for making mistakes. Children need to be invited to feel their feelings and to put words on them so that they can learn gently how not to be impulsive and controlled by their feelings.

Dysfunctional families, however, respond to the neediness and dependence of a child in ways that interfere with the development of authenticity (Figure 2-2). In the dysfunctional family, children are to be seen and not heard. They do not feel free to make mistakes, but feel that if they are not "right" they will be called stupid. "Children are virtuous when they are meek, agreeable, considerate and unselfish."[5,p.7] Adults assume the role of authoritarian masters, intent on breaking the child's will at any cost, or they tend to absent themselves totally from parenting, escaping in alcohol, work, mental illness or travel. Children, who think of their parents as perfect, soon begin realizing that they are not free to act natural, or to be a child, and so adopt another way of being, usually that of comforting and nurturing the parent. The child thus becomes parent to the parent. As a result, a false self emerges in the child. According to psychologist Alice Miller,[6] the persistent denial of the true self and true feelings takes its toll in the development of the coping mechanisms of depression or feelings of grandeur, neither of which is facilitative to a realistic view of the world or to healing.

Health Professionals' Self Esteem

It has been said that many people enter the health professions for a variety of poor, though unconscious, reasons. Among those reasons might be a need to be depended upon, a need to control people and a need to get one's natural attention and affection needs met. Some may be looking for emotional healing themselves by way of making life easier for others. Few people are conscious of these motives, however. Nonetheless they act in ways that are responsive to their unconscious needs and thus do things that are harmful, in the long run, to patients and are contrary to the healing process. These are the characteristics of "early helpers."

Dysfunctional families breed early helpers. One example of a dysfunctional family is the family where one or both parents are addicted to alcohol. It is estimated that "28 to 34 million children and adults in the United States today grew up or are presently being raised in alcoholic homes."[6] The literature that has developed from the Adult Children of Alcoholics (ACOA) movement in the United States has shed needed light on the distorted world view of the adult who grew up in a home where one or more of the parents were not able or willing to parent. This circumstance encourages the development of the "false self," stifles the successful resolution of the tensions described by Erikson, and contributes to chronic low self-esteem and feelings of being, if not "very bad," never good enough. All children experience shame, but children in dysfunctional families take on shame as part of their identity. Children in dysfunctional families are never free to be children; they have to be grown-up and helpful. And it seems as if, since this is a difficult task indeed, they're always doing something wrong. Shame is different from guilt. Whitfield[5] describes shame as "the uncomfortable or painful feeling that we experience when we realize that part of us is defective, bad, incomplete, rotten, phony, inadequate or a failure." (p. 46) Thus guilt says, "I made a mistake"; shame says, "I am a mistake."

Self-esteem can be viewed as the extent to which we are able and willing to "own" our essential goodness (our true self) in the face of our own incompleteness or lack of perfection. More than simply self-acceptance, self-esteem includes pride in the promise of ongoing growth and change with maturity, the hope of a richer, more peaceful and congruent life as a result of honest, day-to-day struggle. Children reared in dysfunctional families feel the shame of never being quite good enough rather than confidence and pride in doing the best they can. Because they were ridiculed and punished just for being, they grow up repressing hurtful feelings, thus believing they had a marvelous family life as a child. But underneath the repressed feelings lie severe self-esteem problems that must be admitted and talked about in order for one to identify the "lenses." Feelings of shame must be identified and confronted, and replaced with a more humane, realistic acceptance of one's own imperfections and essential goodness.

Parental dysfunction may or may not be due to alcohol or drug dependence. The critical factor seems to be how well the parent was present for the growing child in such a way as to encourage the natural curiosity of the child, the natural desire to learn and grow and explore the world, how well the parent nurtured and protected the child and how "safe" and free from potential harm the child felt.[5] When the parent absents him or herself from those responsibilities, for whatever reason (drug dependence, workaholism, depression or mental illness, absence of a good model for parenting) the child starts parenting the parent, and an "early helper" emerges. A common description given by children from dysfunctional families is that they feel that they were a burden, they feel that they were being "bad" when they simply showed natural curiosity or asked questions. In fact, it was their very existence that seemed to bring unending pain and suffering to their family.

Children are not meant to be parents. When they take on this role, they take on a "false" self, and authentic feelings of curiosity, fear and need become repressed, covered by feigned feelings of bravery and affection in an attempt to please the needy parent. Common characteristics that materialize from the distorted world view and false view of the self that then emerge include:

- Fear of losing control
- Fear of feelings that seem overwhelming
- Fear of conflict
- Fear of abandonment
- Fear of becoming alcoholic or drug dependent
- Fear of becoming dependent on another person for survival
- Overdeveloped sense of responsibility
- Feelings of guilt and grief
- Inability to relax and have fun spontaneously
- Harsh self-criticism
- A tendency to lie, even when it's not "necessary"
- A tendency to let one's mind wander, to lose track of a conversation, to figuratively "leave the room."
- Denial and/or the tendency to create reality the way you want it to be, rather than the way it is
- Difficulties getting close to people, with intimacy
- Feelings of vulnerability, of being a victim in a harsh world
- Compulsive behavior, tendency to become addicted to things that alter mood
- Comfort with taking charge in a crisis; panic if you can't "do" something in a crisis.
- Confusion between love and pity
- Black and white perspective—all good or all bad
- Internalizing—taking responsibility for others' problems
- Tendency to react rather than act
- Experiencing stress related illnesses
- Overachievement

And, in spite of all of the above, a marvelous ability to survive and cope.[7] Children from dysfunctional families are the "heroes" in health care, the ones who, at great personal sacrifice, go above and beyond the call to fix things for everyone else and are praised and admired for it. They thrive on rescuing others and on creating order out of chaos. And, very often, these are the people others admonish to "lighten up," for they take every aspect of their lives very seriously.

As Miller points out, having a world view that necessitates the above coping behaviors, the behaviors of a "false self" not the "true self," inevitably leads to depression and often to the desired comfort of addiction as well.[6] Addictive behavior is repeated, habitual behavior designed to bring comfort and to take attention away from experiencing what appear to be the negative, intense feelings of the "true self" that attempt to break through in a given situation. For all the comfort that the addiction brings, the dependence it brings on chemicals (often depressants), on experienced "highs" or on a kind of numbness simply reinforces a denial and continues to reinforce the "false self," making the authentic or "true self" even more difficult to locate. And whenever the true self is blocked, our life energy, our authenticity and our capacity to truly respond to the question, "Who am I?" are blocked. We cannot grow and become who we were created to be. We are stuck like a mouse on an exercise wheel.

Co-dependence

For many young people, addictive impulses are focused not only on drugs and alcohol, but on another person, a potential source of affection to help ease the pain of never feeling as if one received enough authentic recognition, affection and unconditional love as a child. Discomfort emerges when one nervously admits that he or she cannot live without the other person, the dependency has become so great. Since the true self of the person has been lost long ago, it is the false self that has "fallen in love" and proceeds to do its best to please the other, indeed, to live for the other, much as it did for the parents. This phenomenon of living for (being addicted to) the happiness and well-being of another person is termed "co-dependence." In fact, codependence is experienced with more than just a person. It has been described as ". . .an exaggerated dependent pattern of learned behaviors, beliefs and feelings that make life painful. It is a dependence on people and things outside the self, along with neglect of the self to the point of having little self-identity."[5,p.29] The person demonstrating co-dependent behavior looks *outside* himself or herself to discover what he or she wants, needs, believes in, for identity, security, power and belonging. They look outside themselves to feel whole, to get what is missing inside. The co-dependent person often says "yes" when he/she means "no."

Greeting cards do us a great disservice when they express this pathological view with such sloppy sentimentality, as "Even before I knew what my needs were, you were there to help me. You alone taught me the meaning of true love." These are left over fragments, memories of immature needs from our totally dependent infant. Adults must mature beyond destructive dependence on others to develop autonomy, self-control and interdependence on others.[8,p.18] One's identity, power, self-worth and individuality must be experienced as coming from within.

The Need To Know Ourselves

The mature healing professional must know him or herself well; he or she must be aware of behaviors that will result in harmful dependence on patients for getting personal needs for intimacy met. The end goal of all healing is the restoration of independent function for the highest and deepest quality of life possible for the patient. Patients who depend on us for this function never feel able to make it on their own. We foster this destructive dependence when we, ourselves, depend on our patients to meet our needs for attention, affection and/or power and authority.

Self-awareness helps us to identify if our lenses need resetting, cleaning or replacing. It is very difficult to help others effectively if we need help ourselves. Help is available, through the insights gained in this course, through reading the excellent literature now available for those who grew up in dysfunctional families, from counseling, participation in stress groups and in 12-step groups such as Al Anon, Overeaters Anonymous, Alcoholics Anonymous and Adult Children of Alcoholics (ACOA) groups that meet in all the major cities in the United States. The goal of seeking help is always to become acquainted with the true self that was repressed many years ago. In this process, one gains insight into the distortion of his or her lenses, and then often, for the first time as an adult, clearly discerns that there are choices in behavior and that many of the choices one has habitually made in the past have contributed to a chronic feeling of chaos and victimization. Another goal would be to identify negative shame-based beliefs and replace them with more accepting, cosmic beliefs as described in Chapter One.

The groups listed above were formed by people who realized that compulsive behavior and addictions serve to blunt one's awareness of the true self. In order to rid oneself of addictions, support is necessary. These groups are devoted to helping people heal from their addictive behavior and live authentic and genuine lives in the search for the true self, lost long ago in an effort to cope with the unfair stress of childhood.

Self-Awareness Through Action

The exercises for this chapter are designed to help you review your family history, your growth and development, the messages you received and the values you adopted from growing up in your particular setting and circumstances. Try to withhold judgment on what you remember and experience. Remember, feelings are; they exist. Feelings are neither bad nor good, appropriate nor inappropriate; they just are. However, what we *do* with our feelings, how we respond to them is open to our evaluation and choice. Being aware of our feelings is the first step. No family is perfect, and parents often parent the way they were parented. Use these exercises to gain insight into your experience, and to set goals for your personal growth that will help you become a mature healing professional.

Conclusion

The next chapter will discuss values in more depth. We develop our values initially by learning what to value from significant people in our lives, but a value cannot be said to be our own until we accept it for ourselves and act on it. In your journal reflect on your values that you "caught" from significant people in your life. How many of them can you say you have truly reflected upon or tested and have adopted as your own? Do you hold any values that would be perceived as negative? By whom? How does that make you feel?

References

1. Piaget, J: *The Construction of Reality in the Child.* New York, Basic Books, 1954.
2. Bradshaw, J: *Bradshaw on: The Family.* Deerfield Beach, FL, Health Communications, Inc., 1988.
3. Erikson, EH: *Identity, Youth and Crisis.* New York, WW Norton, 1968.
4. *Identifying Successful Families: An Overview of Constructs and Selected Resources.* Washington, DC, Department of Health and Human Services, 1990.
5. Whitfield, CL: *Healing the Child Within.* Baltimore, The Resource Group, 1986.
6. Miller, A: *The Drama of the Gifted Child.* New York, Basic Books, 1981.
7. Malone, M: Dependent on disorder. *MS Magazine,* 15:50, February, 1987.
8. Greenberg, LS, Johnson, SM: *Emotionally Focused Therapy for Couples.* New York, The Gruilford Press, 1988.

exercises

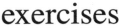
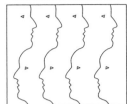

1. Magic Carpet Ride

This exercise is best carried out with the instructor reading the instructions to a group. It is intended to help participants remember what it was like as they were growing up in their families. The magic carpet is a symbol for a ride back into time and memory. Thus, this is a type of guided imagery exercise followed by personal reflection on the content which concludes with a group discussion where participants are able to share with one another, at their own level of comfort, what insights they gained.

Instructor:

"So, sit back in your chairs, feet flat on the floor, and breathe deeply three times, each time feeling more and more relaxed. Concentrate on your breathing, have your mind go blank as you focus on the air going in through your nostrils, and back out through your mouth. With each breath you feel more and more relaxed. (Pause)

I want you to go back in time to when you were a little child, probably in elementary school." (Pause)

"You are inside your house, with your family all gathered together; your parents are there, or those who reared you, and any brothers and sisters are also there." (Pause)

"People are having a conversation." (Pause)

"What are they talking about?" (Pause)

"Now ask them to stop talking for a second because you want to ask each of them an important question. Starting with the adults, ask each one, in turn, to tell you something about you. You're so, what? Listen carefully to the descriptions each gives you and pay attention to the feelings each person seems to display as each answers your question." (Pause for two or three minutes)

"As you get ready to leave the group, say goodbye to each person and come gently forward in time to the present, opening your eyes slowly as you return." (Pause)

"Before talking, write down the names of each person with whom you spoke, then jot down what each told you about yourself, and the feeling or attitude conveyed in that message." (Pause for two or three minutes)

"Now choose one person to share your experience with. Remember, your fantasy was a very private adventure. Some of what you remembered you may decide to keep private. You choose, carefully, the extent to which you want to reveal things about yourself and your family." (Pause five minutes for discussion in two's)

"Now return to your written comments. Search each message for the values that underlie each. For example, if you heard from your mother, "You're so messy! I wish you'd clean up your room," you might discern that she values neatness or obedience to her values. "You're so helpful," naturally leads one to the value of helping or perhaps altruism, unless said with sarcasm. Then search for the message behind the message. Perhaps what was meant was, "I wish you'd stop interfering in my life by always trying to do things for me."

Large Group Discussion

List and discuss various messages and feelings. How many heard essentially negative messages about themselves? How many essentially positive? How many half and half?

How many people live up to the description heard from one or both parents? Negative or positive?

Discuss values inferred from messages.

Conclusion

Record what you learned and felt about the exercise in your journal. Explore the impact that the messages you heard have on your current self-esteem. How do you feel about yourself today, in general? How does that relate to the messages heard? Was this exercise a positive one or a negative one for you? What made it so?

2. Family Genogram

Draw your genogram for at least three generations (Figure 2-1). Label anything which seems important to you. Try to identify any addictions, family tension or conflict or incidents of children parenting their parents.

What patterns emerge? What do you now know about yourself that you failed to see before? What stories are important enough to be handed down? Who/what is the family proud of? What secrets does the family hide from others?

Discuss your genogram with 2 other people in your class that you choose. Each of you should take 5 minutes to describe the people represented, and 25 minutes to discuss the family dynamics as you understand them.

Perhaps questions came up for you about various family members' lives and habits. Write to relatives asking them to fill in the missing pieces to help you better understand your heritage. Try to locate pictures of yourself with other family members from long ago.

Remember, with this exercise in particular, the importance of confidentiality. Nothing revealed should ever leave the classroom. Be worthy of the trust placed in you as others take the risk of discussing private and sensitive material with you.

Journal about your feelings and your awareness from this exercise. Can you identify behaviors that you've developed from your family that may interfere with mature healing? Comment on any, and problem solve ways in which you might be able to work through those behaviors.

A genogram is a map of a family for several generations. It is a very useful picture that reveals multigenerational patterns. An example of a genogram is shown here.

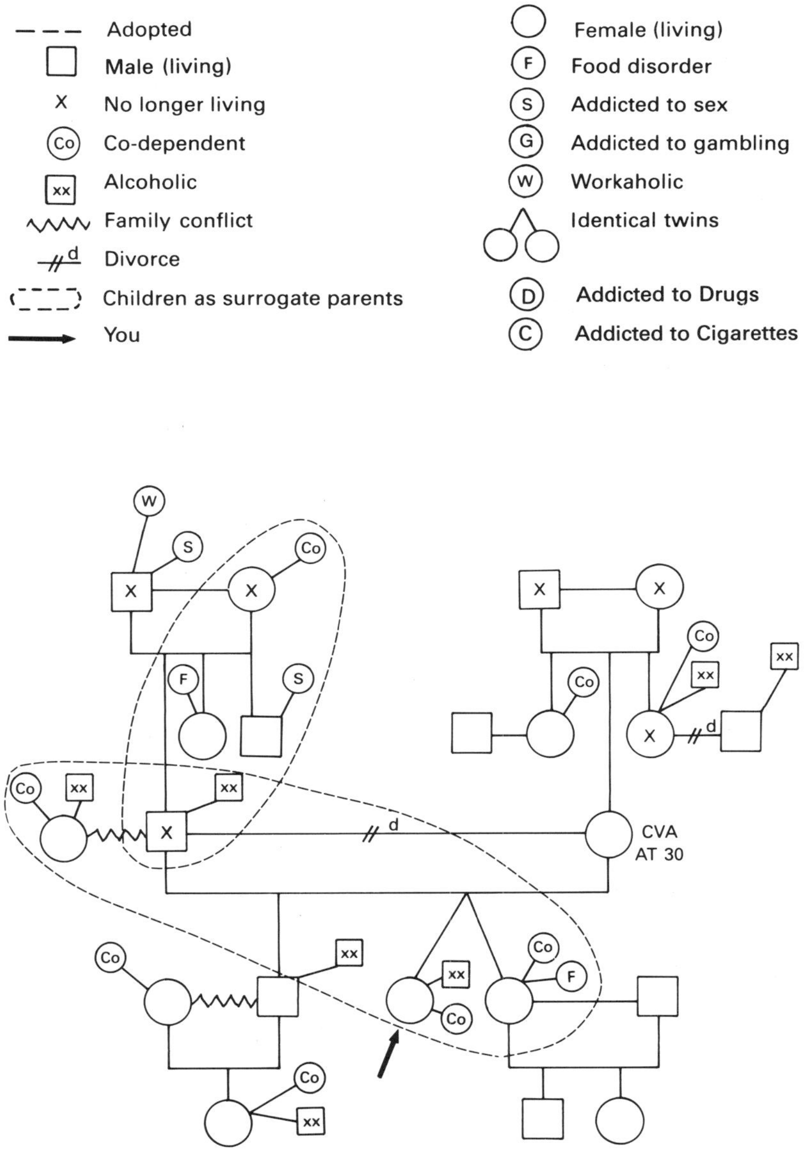

Figure 2-1. Family Genogram

3. Value Boxes

Figure 2-2 is a diagram of eight boxes surrounding a circle that represents you. Each box represents a significant person in your life. Envision a person that corresponds to the descriptor at the top of each box and place that person's initials in the upper right corner. If there is no one who meets that description right now in your life, cross out the descriptor and simply put another important person's initials there. One person should not appear in two boxes.

Now list four or five things you perceive each person would want you to value. What do they count on you for? What demands do they place on you? What do they want you to do, think, be? What do they want you to value?

Now look for similarities from various people. Is there a value that is repeated often? List it below the diagram to the right as a recurring value.

Underline each value that you want for yourself, and place those values in the *center circle*.

Now list the conflict areas to the lower left of the diagram. What do others want for you that you do not desire?

What values seem *most important* to you?

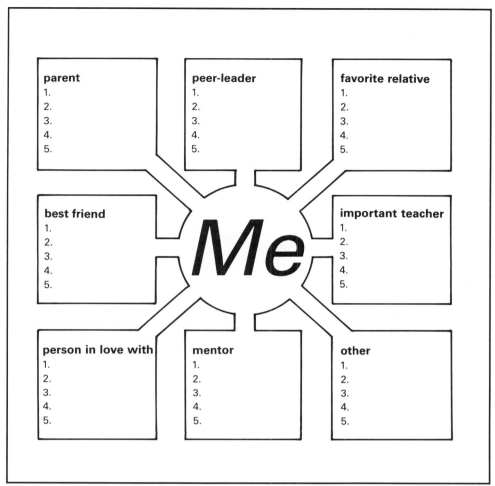

Figure 2-2. Values of Significant Others.

Value Conflicts   **Recurring Values**

chapter three

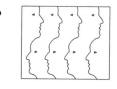

VALUES AS DETERMINANTS OF BEHAVIOR

Objectives

1. To define and examine personal and professional values and to explore the role they play in determining behavior.
2. To emphasize the importance of critical thinking or reflection to the formation of one's values.
3. To examine the values that underlie behaviors that interfere with healing, and those that enhance healing.
4. To distinguish between being morally aware and morally conscious.
5. To distinguish between nonmoral values and moral values.

The process of professional socialization is a process of growth, of becoming a professional person. Ideally that growth is holistic and permeates our selves at deep levels. We realize we've grown, we've learned, when we can observe changes in our behavior. Most obviously, we know more as we become professional. We incorporate an entire new body of knowledge and skill and use much of it daily in our professional care. But we also develop different attitudes and values as we grow professionally. In other words, professional growth involves changes in our knowledge, our skills and our attitudes, values and beliefs.

All people, after a certain age, can be said to have values. Some of those values you've examined in Chapter Two. Consequently, you're now more aware of some of the values you learned and adopted or "introjected" from your family. It is very appropriate for family members to help us grow as children by teaching us what to believe and value when we are too young to choose critically for ourselves. Babies are not born with values. We appreciate this when we eat at a restaurant with a four-year-old who has not yet been socialized adequately and runs around the room playfully throwing food at people.

Sometimes we introject the values of our parents so completely that we don't even know what we value or why. The story is told of a young couple starting life together cooking a special ham dinner for guests. As one partner prepared the roast, he cut the two ends of the ham off before putting it in the oven. His wife chided him for wasting so much meat, and he defended himself by saying that his mother taught him always to cut the ends off. "Why?" she asked. He responded that he didn't know, but he thought it was very important; probably something to do with the proper cooking and circulation of juices.

The next time they visited his parents' home, the new wife asked her husband's mother about cutting the ends off the ham. "Oh, yes," she replied; "My mother always taught me to do that. It's critical to the cooking of the meat."

Still not satisfied, Grandmother was called on the phone. "Grandma, tell our new daughter-in-law why it's so important to cut the ends of the meat off the ham before cooking it!"

Grandma replied, "Oh, that old trick. It's just a habit I got into. When I was first married, we didn't have a big enough pot to fit the meat in, so I just trimmed the ends. After awhile, it just became a habit, I guess."

And so it is with some of the values we "catch" from our parents, without thinking about them. Cutting off the ends of ham is not a good example of value based behavior, but the analogy is important. A clear definition of value based behavior follows shortly.

Carl Rogers'[1] research indicated that immature people, in an attempt to gain or hold love, approval, and esteem, place the locus of evaluation of values on others. They learn to have a basic distrust for direct experiencing as a valid guide to appropriate behavior. They learn from others what values are important, and adopt them as their own, even though they may be widely discrepant from personal experience. Because these introjected values are not based on genuinely experienced personal feelings, they tend to be fixed and rigid, rather than fluid and changing.

Rogers[1] disclosed a list of what he termed the commonly adopted or "introjected" values and their associated beliefs found very often in the subjects from the United States that he studied in the 1950s and 60s:

1. Sexual desires are mostly bad. Source: parents, teachers, the church.
2. Disobedience is bad. To obey is good; to obey without question is better. Source: parents, teachers, the church, the military.

3. Making money is the highest good. Sources: too numerous to mention.
4. Aimless, exploratory reading for fun is undesirable and lazy. Source: teachers, the educational system.
5. Abstract art is good. Source: "the sophisticated people."
6. Communism is all bad. Source: the government.
7. To love your neighbor is the highest good. Source: parents, the church.
8. Cooperation and teamwork are preferable to acting alone. Source: companions.
9. Cheating is clever and desirable. Source: the peer group.
10. Coca-cola, chewing gum, electric refrigerators and automobiles are utterly desirable. Source: advertisements. (This is still reinforced by people in many parts of the world.)

Clearly this list reveals that commonly held values reflect the cultural mores of the time. How might this list change for the 90s? What do you project commonly held social values will be for the early part of the 21st century?

Defining Values

What is a value? Values have been defined in many ways, but in general, the term value refers to an operational belief which one accepts as one's own and which determines behavior. Morrill[2] is far more specific, however, and defines values as:

- standards and patterns of choice that guide persons and groups toward satisfaction, fulfillment, and meaning.
- constructs that orient choice and shape action.
- concepts which call forth thought and conduct that have worth, that lead at least under the right conditions, to the fulfillment of human potential or to the discovery of a variety of types and levels of meaning.
- concepts which are not themselves beliefs or judgments but come to expression in and through thought
- concepts which are not themselves feelings or emotions, but they inevitably involve desires and fears; cannot be defined as deeds, but are always mediated through specific acts.

Thus values orient our choices, and inspire our actions. And since this is a text devoted to developing appropriate professional ways of being, it becomes critical to examine and clarify the values you now hold in relation to the values that form ethical and sensitive professional care giving.

Values Versus Needs

Values can be distinguished from needs, which also influence our behavior. If I am thirsty, without thinking much about it, I get something to drink. Needs push us into behaving in certain predictable ways. A theory of human behavior based upon a hierarchy of needs has been outlined in detail by psychologist Abraham Maslow.[3] But for behavior to be value based, I must reflect upon the choices I have and act according to my reflection. Thus, need behavior is more automatic and driven, whereas value based behavior takes place upon reflection.[4] Implied in this distinction is the idea that value based behavior is more mature, less impulsive, especially when compared to behaviors that are based on the more basic or lower level needs.

Clearly, cutting off the ends of the ham does not represent value based or reflective behavior, but represents an introjected behavior based on the tendency to distrust one's own experience as a guide. Perhaps the value underlying this behavior was to follow the example of elders in spite of logic. Indeed, two generations of the family distrusted their own experience! And so it goes in our families.

Moral Versus Nonmoral Values

The professional socialization process requires the clarification and prioritization of currently held values, and the adoption of new values that are consistent with the values of the profession. Deciding how to prepare ham or what clothes to wear to a party is a decision-making process of a different sort than deciding whether a patient is a good candidate to receive an above-knee prosthesis. The differences are important. The first category is an example of personal choice or preference; the second is a professional decision. Both personal and professional choices can be based on reflection of values, but professional choices are not the same as value preferences. The first is a choice that bears little consequence for the chooser if the less-than-best decision is made. However, the decision about the prosthesis has profound consequence for another person if the less-than-best decision is made.[6]

Values that lead to personal preference are termed *nonmoral values;* values that have to do with the way we relate to and interact with fellow human beings are termed *moral values.*[5] Moral values such as compassion, trust, justice, honesty, love, confidentiality, and faithfulness to one's professional colleagues form the heart of a profession's value structure. Moral values take on more importance than value preferences, and must be regarded with greater seriousness because the needs of human beings are more important than what food or music or hair style we prefer.

Professional Values

There are times when the behavior of health professionals comes into direct conflict with patients' behavior. The values that the profession espouses, for example, in its Code of Ethics, and the behavior observed in many hospitals often seem far removed from each other. Often the behavior exhibited in conflict situations is not value based, or reflective, but impulsive and defensive.

Values conflicts are always rich in their lessons for learning, though many of us shy away from them because we are afraid of doing the wrong thing. In tense times most of us want someone to "tell us what to do."

A moral dilemma exists when we have difficulty choosing which value should have priority. Chapter Four focuses on the examination of ethical dilemmas and their resolution, but a brief example here will illustrate this point. Respect for life is the central value for advocates of a woman's right to choose abortion as well as for those opposed to abortion. The difference in opinion and belief of these two groups is not the value of life, but the importance of the mother's life over the fetus' life. The anti-abortionists claim the primacy of the fetus' life above all considerations; the reproductive-freedom advocates claim the primacy of the mother's choice for the quality of her life and resist outside interference with her right to choose.[6] Likewise, those who favor capital punishment value the lives of those who might become victimized over the life of the dangerous person.

The set of moral norms adopted by a professional group to direct value-laden choices in a way consistent with professional responsibility is termed a Code of Ethics. One might follow the code without internalizing it, introjecting it just as one did in younger years with parents' values. For a code of ethics to function as a set of professional values, one must reflect on it and decide that it, indeed, forms a values complex around which one is willing to organize professional choices. Thus, as stated previously, reflection is necessary to the internalization of values to make them truly one's own, whether personal or professional. Those who make the smoothest transitions into professional practice are likely to be those whose personal values and priorities greatly overlap with the values inherent in their chosen professional practice. Given that one's basic human survival needs are met, the more one reflects on one's choices and upon which choices result in the good and meaningful life, the more one is apt to experience consistent reward from choices made.[6]

Values That Detract From a Therapeutic Presence

Often patients end up needing the help of rehabilitation professionals because of impulsive, poor choices reflecting an immature and inconsistent set of values that have been introjected, but not clarified or claimed as one's own. An example might be the young man who comes to physical therapy needing relief from low back pain incurred from lifting a heavy railroad tie while showing off in front of some young women and men he decided he needed to impress. Many patient problems in movement and function are not the result of "fate," but result from a lifetime of choices that reveal little attention or value to behaviors that preserve physical and emotional health. Thus, it sometimes becomes difficult to avoid becoming judgmental, and as professionals, we sometimes feel resistance to treating people who have not taken good care of themselves and have become, for example, obese, or are chronic smokers.[6]

Professional ethics demand that, when a feeling of criticism and negative judgment of a patient occurs, we must be aware of it and consciously work to not let it interfere with our commitment to compassionate, quality care. Common behaviors that reveal difficulty in this task include the following.

1. Acting cool or aloof, obviously paying more attention to other patients. Underlying value: prejudice or indifference.
2. Overlying criticizing the patient so that he or she feels as if nothing is right. Underlying value: prejudice, perfectionism, rigidity.
3. Treating the patient as an object rather than a person with feelings of pain, worry and insecurity. Underlying value: depersonalization.
4. Treating the patient as if he or she were a child, incapable of understanding or making wise choices. Underlying value: patronizing, adopting an air of condescension.
5. Being unable or unwilling to help the patient in treatment; leaving the patient alone most of the time. Underlying value: indifference or prejudice.
6. Making fun of the patient in his or her presence and/or behind his or her back. Underlying value: depersonalization.
7. Telling others things the patient shared in confidence. Underlying value: breaking confidentiality.
8. Refusing to let the patient work on his or her own; constantly supervising and instructing. Underlying value: fostering dependence. Getting own need to be needed met from patients.
9. Guessing what is best to do. Refusing to find correct and best treatment alternatives. Acting on habit. Underlying value: refusing to recognize and act based on one's own limits of knowledge.
10. Always fitting the patient in as if everything else is more important. Underlying value: selfish interest over needs of patients.
11. Refusing to listen to patient's story of pain and difficulties dealing with pain and dysfunction. Underlying value: importance of defending one self against personal feelings of fear and insecurity around pain and possible addiction.[6]

Most of us would read this list of behaviors and say to ourselves, "I'd never act like that!" But in fact, as much as we would not ever want to act in ways that interfere with healing, when we are unclear of our values, or, more important, when we are not in touch with our feelings, when we don't know ourselves, we often end up doing and saying things, especially under stress, that we regret later. These regretful behaviors stem, in part, from impulsive and immature needs to be spontaneous and egocentric, and arise from feelings of criticism, and the judgment that our patients don't deserve our help. Or perhaps they grow out of unrecognized fears such as not knowing the right thing to do. Perhaps they stem from not having clarified the values underlying a therapeutic presence.

The Values That Reinforce Healing

Essential to a "therapeutic use of self" is the capacity to feel compassion for those who need our help. Compassion is quite different from pity, wherein I feel sorry for this poor person (and secretly feel smug and am thankful that this is not my problem). Compassion in a mature health professional is a value that is fueled with imagination and the ability to envision what is possible from the other person's perspective. When we truly value our patients as human beings, we express behavior based on moral values that enhance healing, such as sincere and active listening, a desire to treat patients as adults, in charge of their own lives and capable of making wise and appropriate decisions for themselves. We treat what they say with confidence and respect; we attend to them with interest and obtain their informed consent for therapeutic procedures. We convey to them that their choice to come to us was well-founded, and that we will help within clearly set boundaries and expectations. In other words, we work to be able to sincerely feel genuine positive regard for all of our patients and relate to each with sensitivity to their uniqueness.

When we become professionals, we gain many things, but we also give up some things. One of the things we give up is the right to walk away from people we would rather not treat. What patient would be your most dreaded? Would it be the rapist? The child abuser? The alcoholic? The person who is HIV positive or has AIDS? When we judge our patients, we can't help but treat them as less than human. What is required is a sense of oneness with all human beings, regardless of the mistakes they may have made. Deciding that the mistakes you have made are far less "evil" only distances you from your patient.

As professionals we also give up the right to say whatever we feel at any moment. We give up the right to speak and act impulsively, and take on the responsibility to act in accordance with the Code of Ethics, or, in similar terms, to act according to the moral values that facilitate healing. No longer may we claim the luxury of spontaneous outbursts or selfish indifference. No longer may we put our own needs before the needs of our patients. No longer may we be run by unclear values or fears that have not yet been examined and resolved.

Professional rehabilitative care requires problem solving that is proactive, based on scientific data and demonstrates a consistent, conscious value of choosing behavior that is conducive to healing. As a professional clinician, you must become an informed reasoner. You must learn to value the systematic gathering of facts and compassionate relating to people who come to you for help. You must value taking the time to reflect on your behavior, and choose to act in ways that reinforce healing. Central to this process is the courage to examine carefully your values and the values of healing and to make a commitment to change behaviors that interfere with effective and compassionate care. Feedback from others is important, but at this point in the text, you are asked to focus on self-examination.

Development of an Ethical Consciousness

We are not born knowing the right thing to do; we develop the ability to solve moral problems in conjunction with cognition. There are three common approaches to teaching children the right thing to do.[2] The most common is the objectivist approach, or legalism, which asserts that to do the right thing is to obey the rules. The "rightness" of the value is within the value itself; therefore, it is always right, for example, to love people, to act justly, honestly, and with compassion. Organized religion teaches this approach to values education. To do the right thing, one should obey the higher authority, do as the Bible says, follow the Torah, or the Ten Commandments, etc. But objectivism offers little help in reconciling the contradictions that can be found in the Bible or resolving the dilemma, for example, between honoring your parents and following your own conscience in developing your career when your choice and the choice your parents would have you make are at odds. Likewise, objectivism fosters the development of a moral belief system based on outside authority. For these reasons it does not adequately serve the purpose of dilemma resolution in health care.

Ethical subjectivism, or values clarification (examined briefly in the exercises) offers an alternative that approaches ethical relativism.[3] Ethical relativism is the view that each person's values should be considered equally valid. Subjectivism suggests that one examine the conflicting values to make sure that each is, indeed, a value. If a belief or idea does not meet true "value" status, it is relegated to a position of less importance than a true value. To satisfy the definition of "value," so Raths and colleagues suggest, a value must satisfy the seven criteria listed in Figure 3-1.[7-9] The content of a value, so important in objectivism, becomes secondary to the process of determining if something is, indeed, a value.[5]

How well does subjectivism assist us in making value based decisions? It probably doesn't make that much difference if one begins treating patients at 8 a.m. or 8:30. People will (and often do) argue the importance of their priorities, but nonmoral values, or value preferences are just that, relative preferences. Moral values present a different story. In fact, moral relativism renders an ethical code meaningless.[5]

Thus in a moral or ethical dilemma in which one must choose between doing the loving thing and following the rules, it does little good to use a subjectivist approach, clarifying if both compassion and justice fit the criteria of a value. What is needed is a way of weighing the relative goodness of each value in the situation. Thus both subjectivism and objectivism fall short of informing us clearly how to decide between two conflicting values, which is the better to choose.

Carol Gilligan[10] and Lawrence Kohlberg[11] both have developed theories that assist us in our task. Their theories each fall under the category of

Choosing one's beliefs and behaviors
1. Choosing freely
2. Choosing from among alternatives
3. Choosing after considering consequences of choice

Prizing one's beliefs and behaviors
4. Prizing and cherishing
5. Publicly affirming when appropriate

Acting on one's beliefs and behaviors
6. Acting
7. Acting repeatedly, showing consistency

Figure 3-1. Rath's Seven Requirements for a Value.

contextualism, in which they assert that, as people develop their ability to think, they also develop their ability to reason about the right or best thing to do in a given situation. This approach to dilemma resolution has been termed contextualism, because the context of the situation provides the key information in deciding the right thing to do *in that situation.* Certain values are, as the objectivists suggest, always going to assume great importance, but the key to resolving the dilemma is to collect all the pertinent data about this particular situation, and then weigh alternatives for the best thing to do, according to the best and most mature debate. How do we discover the most adequate reasoning, the most mature debate? Developmental psychology and philosophy inform us here.

Developmental Aspect of Moral Decision-Making

Developmentalists, in general, assert that as people grow and change, they pass through predictable stages in which new behaviors are formed and stabilized. The maturation process consists of a progression through a series of passages or stages that reflects the increasingly sophisticated changes occurring in a person's nervous system. Thus children are not "little adults" and should not be treated as such, nor be asked to act like adults before they know what that means.

Perhaps the most famous developmentalist, Jean Piaget,[12] suggested that as cognitive abilities develop, the ability to know the right thing to do also develops. Piaget suggested four stages of development of a moral conscience: amoral (ages 0-2), egocentric (ages 2-7), heteronomous (ages 7-12) and autonomous (ages 12 and over) (Figure 3-2). Kohlberg based his work on that of Piaget, and further refined the stages based on research conducted around the world.[11] Kohlberg suggests six stages men and boys go through in developing a mature moral consciousness (Figure 3-2). Earliest and most immature is the punishment and obedience stage in which that which is wrong is that for which I get punished. Figures 3-2 and 3-3 illustrate the progression of stages through stage six, an autonomous stage of knowing the right thing based on a decision of conscience in accord with self-chosen, well-thought-out ethical principles appealing to logical comprehensiveness,

Piaget's Moral Development Model	Kohlberg's Moral Development Model			
	Level	Orientation Stage	Characterized by	Personally stated as
Amoral stage—ages 0 to 2				
Egocentric stages—ages 2 to 7—lacks morality, bends rules and reacts instinctively to environment	*Preconventional*	1. Punishment and obedience orientation	Satisfying one's own needs	I must obey the authority figure or else. . .
		2. Instrumental relativist orientation		
Heteronomous stage—ages 7 to 12—based on total acceptance of a morality imposed by others	*Conventional*	3. Good boy-nice girl orientation	Conformity to social conventions and expectations	I probably should because everyone expects me to.
		4. Law and order orientation	Respect for authority and society's laws	I ought to because of duty to obey the rules.
Autonomous stage—age 12 and over—based on an internalized morality of cooperation	*Postconventional or autonomous*	5. Social contract orientation	Conformity to the ever-changing values and demands of society	I may because of my role in society, but I often question the relative values of society.
		6. Universal ethical principle orientation	My conscience holds me responsible for doing what is right.	I will because I know it is the right thing to do.

Figure 3-2. Comparison of the Stages in Two Models of Moral Development as proposed by Jean Piaget and Lawrence Kohlberg. Used with permission from Francoer, RT. *Becoming a Sexual Person.* New York: John Wiley and Sons, 1982, p 673.

universality and consistence and that flow from the basic principle of justice.[11] When faced with dilemmas, Kohlberg observed that people did not just work out the right answer for themselves by guessing or by trial and error. Rather, depending on their age and maturity, they appealed to a category of reasons outlined in the stages in Figure 3-3. As you can see, both Kohlberg and Piaget believed that children progress from a total abdication to an outside authority to an autonomous stage wherein they make their own choices.

Carol Gilligan,[10] also a contextualist and student of Kohlberg, reacted to the fact that Kohlberg only studied men and boys and then generalized his theory to girls and women. Kohlberg stated that girls and women get

1. **Preconventional Level**
   Child is responsive to cultural rules and labels of good and bad or right and wrong only as they relate to physical consequence of action (reward or punishment).

   Stage 1—Punishment and obedience orientation
   Avoidance of punishment and unquestioning deference to power valued in their own right, not in terms of respect for underlying moral order supported by punishment and authority (Stage 4).

   Stage 2—Instrumental relativist orientation
   Right actions are those that satisfy one's own needs. Reciprocity is not a matter of loyalty or justice, but of "You scratch my back and I'll scratch yours."

2. **Conventional Level**
   Maintaining the expectations of the individual's family, group or nation is valuable in its own right, regardless of consequences.

   Stage 3—Interpersonal concordance or "good boy-nice girl" orientation
   Good behavior is that which pleases others and is approved by them. Behavior is often judged by intention. One earns approval by being "nice."

   Stage 4—"Law and order" orientation
   Right behavior consists of showing respect for authority, following the rules, doing one's duty, and maintaining the given social order for its own sake.

3. **Post-Conventional, Autonomous, Principled Level**
   Clear effort to define moral values and principles that have validity and application apart from authority of groups or other persons holding these principles.

   Stage 5—Social contract, legalistic orientation
   Right actions are defined as those that have been critically examined and agreed upon by the whole society. Emphasis placed on procedural rules for reaching consensus in the face of relativism. Aside from what is constitutionally and democratically agreed upon, what is right is a matter of personal values and opinion. It is possible to change the law when it is to the benefit of society. Outside the law, free agreement and contract are the binding elements of obligation (the "official" morality of the U.S. government and Constitution).

   Stage 6—Universal-ethical principle orientation
   Right is defined by the decision of conscience in accord with self-chosen ethical principles appealing to logical comprehensiveness, universality, and consistency. The basic universal principles are those of justice, of the reciprocity and equality of human rights, and of respect for the dignity of human beings as individual persons, no matter which nationality, race, color, or creed.

Figure 3-3. Kohlberg's Stages of Moral Development.

"stuck" in stage three: Good boy-nice girl orientation that reveals conformity to social expectation, because girls are socialized to stay at home and tend the house, yielding to the decisions of the man in the house. Right is that which pleases others.

Gilligan's work challenges the rigidity of this assumption.[10] In her studies of how girls, college women and housewives, perceive the same set of moral problems outlined by Kohlberg, she reveals that women "appear to frame moral problems in terms of conflicting personal responsibilities rather than conflicting rights and the concept of justice."[10] Thus, as a function of social conditioning, adolescent boys may well focus first on achievement and self-identity, and much later focus on developing a value of intimacy and friendship, while girls do just the opposite. Both genders have the same ability to mature to higher stages of moral conscience; that is, girls and women do not simply stop maturing morally at stage three. However, girls and women seem to mature, not linearly as Kohlberg's scale illustrates, but horizontally, in netlike fashion, favoring the higher importance of relationship over abstract goals such as social justice and achievement.

Moral Awareness Versus Moral Consciousness

To be morally aware is to know what the dictionary says about, for example "compassion," and to be somewhat aware if your behavior fits that description at any given time. To be morally *conscious,* however, is to examine how compassion weaves its way through your behavior, how it influences you in your various decisions, how you feel about compassion with regard to justice, for example, in a moral dilemma. Thus moral consciousness represents a deeper way of knowing and thus a firmer commitment to consistency in moral behavior, or the way we interact with other human beings. The goal of this text is, at the least, to confirm your moral awareness, and ideally, to help stimulate a moral consciousness that is consistent with quality, compassionate health care. Knowing the right thing to do does not guarantee doing the right thing. But it is a major first step. Pellegrino suggests[7] that quick self-examination on the effectiveness of one's therapeutic presence might be accomplished by answering these three questions truthfully:

1. Do I listen and not only respond to, but satisfy the fundamental questions each person who is ill and anxious brings to me?
2. Can I accept the patient for what he or she is, not for what I think he or she should be?
3. Can I handle my authority in a humane way that respects the life and values of the patient?

To be able to answer yes to any of these questions requires that we continue to grow as persons as we become professionals. The value of a lifelong commitment to growth and increasing moral consciousness insures a meaningful and peaceful professional as well as personal life.

Awareness Through Activity

The exercises are designed to help you further analyze important personal values you currently hold, to help you learn which of your values you value most, or what is your highest order value. A visit to a clinic or patient care area where you will be asked to make careful observations of behavior and to comment on the values that seem to underlie it will help sensitize you to the stresses of patient care, and will illustrate various kinds of interactions that take place with patients. Finally, a "forced choice" exercise will pull out some introjected values that you may not even be aware you hold.

References

1. Rogers, C, Stevens, B: *Person to Person—The Problem of Being Human.* Lafayette, California, Real People Press, 1967.
2. Morrill, R: *Teaching Values in College.* San Francisco, Jossey-Bass, 1980.
3. Maslow, A: *Motivation and Personality.* Harper and Row, New York, 1954.
4. Beck, C: A philosophical view of values and value education. In Hennessy, T (ed): *Values and Moral Development.* New York, Paulist Press, 1976.
5. Wehlage, G, Lockwood, AL: Moral relativism and values education. In Purpel, D and Ryan, K (eds): *Moral Education—It Comes With the Territory.* Berkeley, McCutchen, 1976.
6. Davis, CM: Influence of values on patient care: foundation for decision making. In O'Sullivan, S and Schmitz, T: *Foundations of Rehabilitation,* 2nd ed. Philadelphia, FA Davis, 1988.
7. Pellegrino, ED: Educating the humanist physician—an ancient ideal reconsidered. In *Fostering Ethical Values During the Education of Health Professionals.* Proceedings of a conference of the Society for Health and Human Values. Philadelphia, 1975.
8. Davis, CM: The influence of values on patient care. In Payton, OD (ed): *Psychosocial Aspects of Clinical Practice.* New York, Churchill Livingstone, 1986.
9. Simon, SB, Howe, L, Kirschenbaum, H: *Values Clarification—A Handbook for Teachers.* NYC, Hart Publishers, 1972.
10. Gilligan, C: *In a Different Voice.* Cambridge, Harvard University Press, 1983.
11. Kohlberg, L: The cognitive development approach to moral education. *Phi Delta Kappa.* June 1975, pp. 670-677.
12. Piaget, J: *The Construction of Reality in the Child.* New York, Basic Books, 1954.

exercises

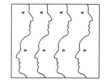

1. Values Clarification Chart

Values shape and orient our choices, and so one way to examine our values is to examine our choices and to see if those choices have been made after reflection. On the next page is a chart that helps you explore things that can be said to be of value to most people. In addition to inquiring about the manner of choosing the item, and its underlying value, the chart, taken from Simon, et al.,[9] also asks us how positive we feel about the item and its value. The Values Clarification theorists claim that, in order to be a true value (as compared to a hope or aspiration or goal), it must meet these seven criteria of choosing, prizing and acting:

Choosing (Table 3-1.)
1. Chosen freely
2. Chosen from among alternatives
3. Chosen after thoughtful consideration

Prizing
1. Cherish it
2. Publicly affirm it

Acting
1. Do something about it
2. Consistently act on it in life as pattern

    A. Complete the chart on your own.

    B. Discuss with one or two other classmates for 10 minutes.

    C. Journal about what you learned.

Table 3–1.
Values Clarification Chart

ITEM	WHAT MAKES IT VALUABLE? UNDERLYING VALUE	CHOOSING 1	CHOOSING 2	CHOOSING 3	PRIZING 1	PRIZING 2	ACTING 1	ACTING 2
1. Something I'm saving money for.								
2. Most important thing I did last year.								
3. Something I quit doing recently.								
4. My dream vacation—no restrictions.								
5. One thing I'm proud of.								
6. A risk I'm glad I took.								
7. Something I learned to do in the past few years.								

2. Values Priority Exercise

Life Planning Handout—Value in Life?

Name _____ Date _____

Age _____ Year in College _____

Years living away from parent's home _____

1. Read through the entire list. This is not a semantics test, so feel free to cross out the definition and add your own if you wish.
2. Circle each items' level of importance to you.
3. After completing item 2 above, pick out and list in the spaces provided the five items that you feel are the most important to you and the five items that are the least important.

ACHIEVEMENT (Accomplishment; results brought by resolve, persistence, or endeavor)
    not very important   important   very important

AESTHETICS (Appreciation and enjoyment of beauty for beauty's sake, in both arts and nature)
    not very important   important   very important

ALTRUISM (Regard for or devotion to the interest of others; service to others)
    not very important   important   very important

AUTONOMY (Ability to be a self-determining individual; personal freedom; making own choices)
    not very important   important   very important

CREATIVITY (Developing new ideas and designs; being innovative)
    not very important   important   very important

EMOTIONAL WELL BEING (Peace of mind, inner security; ability to recognize and handle inner conflicts)
    not very important   important   very important

HEALTH (The condition of being sound in body)
    not very important   important   very important

HONESTY (Being frank and genuinely yourself with everyone)
    not very important   important   very important

JUSTICE (Treating others fairly or impartially; conforming to fact, truth, or reason)
    not very important   important   very important

KNOWLEDGE (Seeking truth, information, or principles for the satisfaction of curiosity)
    not very important   important   very important

LOVE (Want, caring; unselfish devotion that freely accepts another in loyalty and seeks his good)
    not very important   important   very important

LOYALTY (Maintaining allegiance to a person, group, or institution)
    not very important   important   very important

MORALITY (Believing and keeping ethical standards; personal honor, integrity)
    not very important   important   very important

PHYSICAL APPEARANCE (Concern for one's attractiveness; being neat, clean, well-groomed)
    not very important   important   very important

PLEASURE (Satisfaction, gratification, fun, joy)
    not very important   important   very important

POWER (Possession of control, authority of influence over others)
    not very important   important   very important

RECOGNITION (Being important, well-liked, accepted)
    not very important   important   very important

RELIGIOUS FAITH (Having a religious belief; being in relationship with God)
    not very important   important   very important

SKILL (Being able to use one's knowledge effectively; being good at doing something important to me or others)
    not very important   important   very important

WEALTH (Having many possessions and plenty of money to do anything desired)
    not very important   important   very important

WISDOM (Having mature understanding, insight, good sense, and judgment)
    not very important   important   very important

Five Least Important: **Five Most Important:**

Directions: Number 1 = Favorite value of the 5 listed. Transfer numbers to summary table on next page.

The Five-Sort Value Inventory

1. ( ) Achievement
   ( ) Altruism
   ( ) Justice
   ( ) Religious Faith
   ( ) Wealth

2. ( ) Altruism
   ( ) Autonomy
   ( ) Loyalty
   ( ) Power
   ( ) Recognition

3. ( ) Creativity
   ( ) Love
   ( ) Pleasure
   ( ) Recognition
   ( ) Wealth

4. ( ) Aesthetics
   ( ) Justice
   ( ) Pleasure
   ( ) Power
   ( ) Wisdom

5. ( ) Altruism
   ( ) Honesty
   ( ) Love
   ( ) Physical Appearance
   ( ) Wisdom

6. ( ) Achievement
   ( ) Aesthetics
   ( ) Health
   ( ) Honesty
   ( ) Recognition

7. ( ) Achievement
   ( ) Autonomy
   ( ) Physical Appearance
   ( ) Pleasure
   ( ) Skill

8. ( ) Autonomy
   ( ) Emotional Well Being
   ( ) Health
   ( ) Wealth
   ( ) Wisdom

9. ( ) Honesty
   ( ) Knowledge
   ( ) Power
   ( ) Skill
   ( ) Wealth

10. ( ) Achievement
    ( ) Emotional Well Being
    ( ) Love
    ( ) Morality
    ( ) Power

11. ( ) Aesthetics
    ( ) Autonomy
    ( ) Knowledge
    ( ) Love
    ( ) Religious Faith

12. ( ) Aesthetics
    ( ) Loyalty
    ( ) Morality
    ( ) Physical Appearance
    ( ) Wealth

13. ( ) Creativity
    ( ) Health
    ( ) Physical Appearance
    ( ) Power
    ( ) Religious Faith

14. ( ) Health
    ( ) Justice
    ( ) Love
    ( ) Loyalty
    ( ) Skill

15. ( ) Aesthetics
    ( ) Altruism
    ( ) Creativity
    ( ) Emotional Well Being
    ( ) Skill

16. ( ) Emotional Well Being
    ( ) Justice
    ( ) Knowledge
    ( ) Physical Appearance
    ( ) Recognition

17. ( ) Altruism
    ( ) Health
    ( ) Knowledge
    ( ) Morality
    ( ) Pleasure

18. ( ) Morality
    ( ) Recognition
    ( ) Religious Faith
    ( ) Skill
    ( ) Wisdom

19. ( ) Emotional Well Being
    ( ) Honesty
    ( ) Loyalty
    ( ) Pleasure
    ( ) Religious Faith

20. ( ) Achievement
    ( ) Creativity
    ( ) Knowledge
    ( ) Loyalty
    ( ) Wisdom

21. ( ) Autonomy
    ( ) Creativity
    ( ) Honesty
    ( ) Justice
    ( ) Morality

Value Inventory Rating Summary

To summarize the results of the previous exercise, enter the numbers you recorded (for the first set of five) in the first box of each of these values below. Each value occurs five times, so when you are through recording all 21 sets of five, you will have five entries for each value. Add those five numbers across. The Totals column will then give you some ideas of the respective weights you give to the values involved. Remember, the lower the number in the Totals column, the higher that value ranks in your priorities.

						Totals
1. Achievement						
2. Aesthetics						
3. Altruism						
4. Autonomy						
5. Creativity						
6. Emotional Well Being						
7. Health						
8. Honesty						
9. Justice						
10. Knowledge						
11. Love						
12. Loyalty						
13. Morality						
14. Physical Appearance						
15. Pleasure						
16. Power						
17. Recognition						
18. Religious Faith						
19. Skill						
20. Wealth						
21. Wisdom						

Top 3 values:

3. Environmental Crisis

This is another exercise designed to help you learn more about the values you learned at home, some of which you may not have given much thought to, but accept as true and often believe everyone accepts them as true.

The Situation

You are a young health professional in a moderately sized metropolitan hospital which has an entire unit devoted to the care of patients with kidney disease. The Kidney Unit can accommodate five people at a time on dialysis and is the only unit within a 500 mile radius that has dialysis capability. At times there are scheduling difficulties, at which time a committee is called together to help resolve decisions of priority. The committee is made up of health personnel from the hospital and community, and of lay people from the community. You are on that committee.

The community in which you live and work has had a crisis. A toxin has leaked into the water supply for the city and has made over half of the citizens terribly ill. Those most vulnerable to the toxin are people with kidney disease. Ten people lie near death (within one hour) unless their blood is dialyzed. There are only five machines.

The committee has been called together to decide who should receive priority. It is impossible to save the lives of all of the victims, but you must make the decision of which five will be saved.

Your group has only minimal chart information about the ten people and thirty minutes to make the decision. Your group realizes that there is no alternative to making this choice if five people are to be saved. With no decision, *all ten people will die.*

Here is what you know about the ten people:

Bookkeeper, male, 31 years old

Bookkeeper's wife, 30, six months pregnant

Second year medical student, male, militant African American

Famous historian and author, 41 years old, female

Hollywood actress, 50 years old

Biochemist, 35 year old female

Rabbi, 54 year old male

Olympic athlete, shot put, 19 year old male

College student majoring in a health profession other than medicine, female

Owner of a topless bar, 56 year old male, prison record

Instructions

1. Read the situation carefully.
2. Working alone, decide the five people who are to go on dialysis. You have 10 minutes to make your personal decision.
3. At the instructor's signal, join with three others in the

room and, working as a group of four, decide on the five people to receive dialysis. You have only 20 minutes to make your decision. Argue strongly for your ideas and opinions. The future of these people's lives depends on your group decision. Make sure your group is satisfied with the final list. Agree with other group members only if they truly convince you that their idea is better than yours.

4. Decisions by majority vote are not permitted. Every member of your group must agree with, and be committed to, the decision.

5. Group discussion:

At the end of 30 minutes, one member of each group comes forward and places a mark in the data summary box on the blackboard in the front of the room (Figure 3-2).

Discuss as a group:

a) Why you decided on each person. What were the assumptions you made that convinced you and others of the worth of each person's life?

b) What process did you go through to decide? Once you accepted the responsibility for the decision, was it difficult to decide on the final five? Who in the group was most convincing? How vocal were you in arguing for what you felt was right?

c) What values emerged as you decided on the worth of a person's life and the opportunity for that person to continue living? Where did those values come from? When your decision was challenged, were you surprised that someone placed a different value higher than yours? Or did you assume most everyone would agree with you?

d) After reflecting a few minutes, comment on this exercise and what it teaches us about the nature of stereotype, labeling and prejudice. How might this affect our decisions as clinicians?

Journal about what you felt as you completed the exercise and what you learned about yourself with regard to what you believe is true and worthwhile, and what you learned about your style of arguing for what you believe in. What are you feeling?

Did anyone agree that every life has equal value and therefore suggest a lottery? How do you feel about that idea?

Table 3–2.
"Values as Determinants of Behavior"

GROUP	1	2	3	4	5	6	TOTAL
Bookkeeper							
Bookkeeper's wife							
Medical student							
Historian							
Hollywood actress							
Biochemist							
Rabbi							
Athlete							
Health professional student							
Topless bar owner							

4. Clinical Field Trip

This is an exercise designed to deepen your understanding of the nature of health care behavior and, specifically, of patient-clinician interaction. Read over the questions below carefully and then visit a facility where patients are being treated by health professionals from the profession you've chosen. Visit as an observer only, as a "fly on the wall" and carefully make observations from which you'll respond to the question asked. Once the questions are answered, journal about what you learned and felt with this experience.

1. What pleased you about what you saw?
2. What bothered you?
3. How did this experience impact on your choice to be a health professional?

Clinical Interaction Observation

1. Observe the environment. Describe how things are ordered, how things appear, and comment on possible underlying values.
2. Is efficiency a value? How do the patient care professionals perform or function in relation to wise use of time?

The patient/practitioner relationship is one of the major influencing factors affecting the success of treatment. This relationship is based upon the establishment of sound, professional judgment. No two practitioners approach the patient in exactly the same manner. With experience, you will develop your own personal style of rapport. By observing interactions between experienced health professionals and their patients you will be better prepared to form your own approach to patient interaction.

Use the following questions as a guide to direct your attention to specific aspects of patient treatment. You will be concerned primarily with the verbal and nonverbal communication which exists between practitioner and patient.

Attending Skills

1. What did the practitioner do to attend to the patient's personal needs and/or comfort before, during and after treatment?
2. How did the practitioner maintain the patient's dignity during treatment?
3. Did the practitioner seem to really listen to the patient's description of his or her illness/disability as it is "lived" by that person?

Communication Skills

Nonverbal Behavior

1. Did the practitioner exhibit any personal mannerisms/behavior which might have added to or detracted from gaining the patient's confidence?
2. Could you add and explain why any additional behaviors might have been effective?
3. Was the practitioner a good listener? What behaviors make you say that?
4. Did the practitioner maintain eye contact while talking with patients? If not, did it seem to detract?
5. Were practitioner and patient at the same eye level for most of the time? Comment.

Verbal Behavior

1. Describe and comment on the practitioner's voice quality as he or she communicated with patients (soft-spoken, brusk, rapid, etc.).
2. How did the practitioner seem to motivate the patient? Was the method effective?

Summary

What impressed you most about your visit?
What impressed you least?
What did you learn that you didn't know before?

(Adapted from material developed by Marilyn DeMont, MS, PT, at that time Assistant Professor, Sargent College, Boston University. Currently Director of Professional Development, APTA.)

chapter four

IDENTIFYING AND RESOLVING MORAL DILEMMAS

Objectives

1. To describe professional ethics and to describe an ethical dilemma.
2. To describe the various factors that need to be considered in making a sound ethical decision.
3. To compare discursive or principled ethical reasoning processes with non-discursive aspects of ethical reasoning.
4. To outline the difficulties inherent in using the principles and rules of traditional biomedical ethical reasoning alone in resolving dilemmas.
5. To offer a problem solving approach that incorporates traditional discursive ethical reasoning with non-discursive elements such as story, virtue, discernment, and meta-beliefs.

Ethics is the study of morality. Moral decisions are decisions about what is right and wrong, or better and best to do in a situation. Descriptive ethics discusses the moral systems of a group or culture, normative ethics deals with establishing a moral system that people can use to make moral decisions, and metaethics is the study of the meanings of ethical terms.[1] Bioethics is the application of ethics to health care.

Why should health professionals have to consider the ethical? Practitioners are faced with several decisions each day. Most health professionals place great importance on making sound clinical or therapeutic decisions in their practice. At times, the legal ramifications of a clinical decision become apparent. But seldom do practitioners consider the ethical or moral implications of their decisions unless they come face to face with a difficult moral dilemma, one that is not easy to resolve with confidence.

Whereas clinical decisions are based on weighing and considering facts (for example, given these lab values and these symptoms, the diagnosis seems to be X) moral decisions are based on weighing and considering values, so there is no such thing as a *true* or *false* moral decision. But just as it is highly important for health professionals to make the right clinical decision, it is assumed that practitioners would rather act ethically than not, choosing the highest or best moral alternative in a value laden dilemma.

Clinical decisions, no matter how purely factual they seem, still deal with people making decisions about what is best and true for other people. Few clinical decisions, especially those which deal with alternative treatment choices, are void of a moral component, for most clinical decisions necessitate weighing the value of various outcomes. Different people may place different importance on the values aspects of any decision.[2] Value laden ethical decisions, like factual clinical decisions, are better made if they are made thoughtfully and rationally, not based solely on intuition or the emotion of the moment.

Some ethical decisions are simple to solve. In the same or similar situation, the majority of people would do the same thing. There is often no valid choice involved, for example in deciding between good and evil—refusing to assist, indeed, trying to prevent a depressed person from taking his own life.

More difficult ethical decisions deal with which is better and which is worse—do I continue to treat (and bill) this terminally ill patient even when my treatment is of little benefit, but my visit seems to make a big difference in the quality of his day to day existence? Not everyone would decide the same. This might be seen to be a struggle between the ethical principles of beneficence (contribute to the good of each patient) and distributive justice (just distribution of limited resources to those who would benefit most).

The most difficult ethical decisions are dilemmas wherein we are faced with choosing two mutually exclusive goals. The choice of the right thing to do not only is very unclear, acting on one moral conviction means breaking another.[1] For example, as a physical therapist, if I act on behalf of my patient recovering from a stroke, but in a plateau stage, and document that he is still progressing with physical therapy, I am not telling the truth, for he has gone into a stage where progress is not obvious each day. However, if I tell the truth, the best interests of my patient are compromised, for the third party reimbursement will be withdrawn and he will not be able to pay for therapy and then, in my professional opinion, he will regress. This illustrates a dilemma where beneficence, acting in the best interest of my patient means breaking a moral conviction to tell the truth. Which is the higher moral alternative? How do I decide?

Some would say that the most difficult of all moral decisions in health care have to do with allocation of scarce resources. Who deserves to receive help and on what do we base our decision?[2] The above situation may illustrate the third party payors' reply to the question of distributive justice, that is, only those who are showing regular change—either improvement or decline—should be reimbursed for physical therapy services.

When faced with an ethical decision, what do we do? We could ignore it, we could follow our ideas or perceptions of "current custom," (what "everyone else would do in this situation"), we could ask our superior what to do, we could search for a policy that speaks to our problem, or a rule to follow, we could do what feels emotionally best or right, we could follow our perception of the dictates of our religion, we could follow our perception of the dictates of our family rules, or we could apply traditional methods of ethical dilemma resolution in the search for the best moral alternative.[2]

This last suggestion is advocated in bioethics, of course, but unfortunately, many health professionals choose one of the former alternatives and "hope for the best." Ethical dilemma resolution has not received the attention in professional curricula that clinical decision making has received. Many health professional educators feel very uncomfortable teaching students how to decide the best moral alternative, for there is no one principle that binds us, there is no absolute dictum against which we can measure the adequacy of our moral choice as being best.

Bioethics Versus Everyday Ethics

What issues come to your mind when we speak of bioethics or health care ethical decisions? The press favors reporting life and death moral dilemmas that deal with issues that reflect the increasing impact of high technology on health care: organ transplants, fetal tissue research, euthanasia and abortion, for example. Granted, these ethical dilemmas are important, and we all benefit from studying the ethical treatment given these issues from ethicists who help direct us in our own decision making. Our task is to read the various arguments and to decide which argument and conclusion seems to match our own evaluation of the best alternative, both in terms of logical soundness and consistency, and in terms of what we feel in our hearts is the highest moral alternative.

Bioethicists would tell us that our hearts should have nothing to do with this problem solving, for our hearts contaminate our reasoning with subjectivity that cannot be substantiated with logic.[3] This would seem more acceptable if we were robots dealing with robots. Because we are people, health professionals dealing with the every day issues of deciding the best thing to do with people who are our patients and their families, it is impossible for many of us to find comfort solely in the rationalistic discursive resolving of dilemmas according to principles alone. The compelling facts of each situation, our own personal priorities, our personal knowledge of the individuals and situation involved and our own personal integrity developed over time by making decisions and weighing the consequences, will all come into play to help us decide which is the best decision in this particular situation, with the limited information we have in this moment.

Rarely do we deal with the life and death ethical problems of euthanasia day to day. The ethical dilemmas we face day to day have to do with trying to do the best thing for our patients within the organization or institution of health care delivery, created mainly to meet the needs of great numbers of people, not individuals. These dilemmas often have to do with maintaining or improving the quality of a single patient's life. In discussing quality of life in the nursing home, the well known ethicist, Arthur Caplan,[4] says it this way:

> In one sense the disproportion of time and energy spent discussing transplants, artificial hearts, and other issues of high technology, acute care medicine, is appropriate. Matters of when and whether life should be maintained are of fundamental ethical importance, but the seemingly small stakes involved in the nursing home context—setting mealtimes and bedtimes, use of the phone, the right to keep personal property in one's nightstand— should not lull anyone into thinking that daily life in a nursing home lacks either ethical content or importance.

A survey of the most common ethical issues faced by physical therapists in New England reported in 1980 listed issues such as which patients should be treated, the obligations entailed by that decision, who should pay for treatment, and what duties are incumbent on physical therapists as they relate to physicians and other professionals.[5]

Ingredients of a Moral Decision

A moral statement says that, in situation X, person Y should do Z. Thus a moral statement includes: what should be done (Z), who is to do it (Y) and the conditions under which the statement is applicable (X).[2] Most decisions made each day in health care are working decisions based on the facts of the situation. The decision is subject to modification or even reversal when more facts become known. Decisions have to be provisional when each day brings new facts to bear. This is the reality of day-to-day health care. "Our task then," according to Francoeur, "is to collect as much information as possible and then refer to the principles involved and choose the highest or best moral alternative in light of the situation at hand."[6,p.96]

Let's take a look at discursive or principled ethical reasoning and see how it can guide us in deciding the highest or best alternative, and then look at nondiscursive methods that will help us discover our own "metabeliefs" which underlie and influence our final decisions about what truly is right and best in each situation.

Traditional Bioethics

Traditional discursive or principled ethical reasoning requires adherence to four levels of thinking: 1) the *particular ethical decision* will be made by 2) favoring an *ethical rule* which 3) sits within an *ethical principle* which 4) evolves out of an *ethical system.*

Ethical systems grow out of how we tend to view the world, or, in the terminology of Chapter One, how we "set our lenses."[6] We try on and adopt points of view about right and wrong as we're growing up and following the dictates of higher authorities such as our parents and church authorities.

Two ethical systems predominate—1) ends or results oriented systems that say that the best way to decide the right thing to do is to act to bring about the best result, the maximum good, (teleological systems) and 2) duty oriented systems or deontological systems which say that the proper decision should not simply be decided by the results. The highest moral alternative should be situated in principles or rules known to be right whether they serve good ends or not.[2] In sum, in deciding the best thing to do, does the end (commonly the greatest good) most of the time justify the means, or do the means need to be carefully weighed without primary concern for the outcome?

An example of a principle which stems from a teleological or consequential way of looking at an ethical problem (ends are the most important) would be to act so that the greatest good can be brought about for the greatest number. That which is best is that which benefits everyone. Individuals come second to the good of the group. Hospital and nursing home administrators often make decisions based on this principle. Another question that could be asked to weigh the good of an action from this perspective would be, "Would I be satisfied with the consequence of this action if it were done to me?"

On the other hand, duty oriented ethicists would look to ethical principles which are those general and foundational truths, laws or doctrines used by deontological ethicists to generate ethical rules about how to act in certain situations, regardless of the consequences. Many principles exist, and in each situation we appeal to the most relevant and appropriate principle to generate the highest moral action.[6] Previously we described ethical dilemmas that seemed to be related to the principles of beneficence, truth telling and distributive justice. We had to decide whether telling the truth or loyalty to the patient was the highest moral alternative.

Examples of various principles that might be called upon appropriately in health care include the principles of:

1. *autonomy*—freedom to decide, freedom to act, acknowledgment and respect we owe the dignity and autonomy of others. *Informed consent* or the freedom to act on one's own behalf and to implement one's free decision is a right situated in the principle of autonomy.[6]

2. *veracity*—obligation of the health professional and the patient to tell the truth.[6] Moral issues around veracity often concern when and whether to tell the *whole* truth or only part of it. Informing a patient that he has a tumor, and later adding that the tumor is malignant, or cancerous, is one example.

3. *nonmaleficence*—above all, do no harm and in all cases, prevent harm from happening. This principle is often used as the higher alternative of doing everything possible to prolong the life of the patient. But, if a physician decides to give morphine in the final stages of life, a drug that will relieve pain but may shorten life by reducing respiratory capacity, he or she has called upon another principle as the higher moral alternative, that of benefiting the quality of a patient's life by relieving excruciating pain rather than lengthening life.[6]

4. *beneficence*—contribute to the good health and welfare of the patient.[6] At first glance, this may appear to be the same as "do no harm," but the two concepts are, indeed, different.

5. *confidentiality*—respecting the secrets confided by the patient, even after death. At times this becomes difficult because health professionals always deal with more people than just the patient. The rights of the patient often have to be weighed against the rights of others, as in the case where a patient or client confesses he intends to kill someone. To warn the intended victim is to break confidentiality for the higher good of another person's beneficence or autonomy, or right to choose to defend herself.[6]

6. *justice*—this principle is very complex as many theories of justice have been put forth. Common to all of them is the minimal principle that like cases should be treated alike, or equals should be treated equally and unequals unequally. Just distribution of limited resources has become the most critical dilemma in health care in the United States. This is an example of *distributive justice. Compensatory justice* has to do with compensation for wrongs done. (Victims of second hand smoke may ask that they be compensated for their illnesses from the smokers they had lived with.) *Procedural justice* has to do with fairness, as in, "first come, first served." Impartiality is strived for here. A key question then is, do patients who have severe pain, or an immediate life threatening condition move to the head of the line or must they wait their turn?[1,6]

Advantages and Difficulties with the Utilization of Principles

When one is face to face with having to decide which is the highest moral action to take in a given situation, it helps to be freed up from the intensity and confusion of spontaneous feelings. This is true whether we're deciding a "true" biomedical dilemma such as distributive justice—who should be treated and who should not, or a day to day dilemma such as the head nurse who has to decide whether the dying patient on the unit can have a visit from his grandchildren from out of town who arrived after visiting hours were over.

Utilizing a reflective problem solving process that takes into account all of the given facts and uncovers all of the principles and rules that might apply is a way to rise above the subjective moment in an attempt to articulate an objective and defensible rationale for your decision. Trying to discern the *best* rule or principle, or the *highest* moral action is often the most difficult decision, especially when you have limited information and must act right away.

We've stated that a teleologist will adopt the point of view that the facts should be weighed and the action that is best would be the action that benefits the greatest number. (The head nurse decides that the visit of young grandchildren might be disruptive to other patients—the greatest number—and decides not to allow it.)

The duty oriented person will refer to a list of principles and pull out all of those that seem to bear on the case, and weighing the facts, decide which principle is the highest in this situation. (The head nurse decides that beneficence, contributing to the good of the patient, is more important than worrying about future decisions if *all* patients ask for this privilege and the chaos that might result [justice].)

The Difficulties of Principled Decision-Making

Edmund Pellegrino, a well known medical ethicist, asks, "Is there a set of obligations which bind all who practice medicine?"[7,p.192] Is there one rule, or set of rules that health professionals will find almost always is the highest moral alternative in health care? This task of deciding would be made simpler if there were. Put simply, adherence to principles doesn't always work because people disagree about which principles are most acceptable. Gilligan posits that "the way people define moral problems, the situations they construe as moral conflicts in their lives and the values they use in resolving them are all a function of their social conditioning."[6] Thus even recognizing a problem as having an ethical aspect to it has a lot to do with how we were brought up, and how we view the world, how our "lenses are set."

In an excellent attempt to present an alternative philosophical basis for medical practice, Pellegrino and Thomasma[7] suggest three values that are primary in the unique practice of medicine, and rather than depending on arguing from teleological or deontological rules, actions of all health professionals should result from these values:

1. *It is good to be healthy.*
   Ethical axiom—help, or at least, do no harm. Thus when deciding the best thing to do, always do that which helps a person or does no harm.
2. *Individuals have intrinsic value.*
   Ethical axiom—individual care and specially tailored treatment should be given to *each* person. In a conflict, individual obligation usually precedes attention to the larger common good. Also, because of the vulnerability of the patient, ethical actions must be grounded in trust and love; a covenantal relationship occurs between health

professional and patient that goes beyond comradeship, contract or legal cultural expectations. So in deciding the best action for your patient, it is not enough to ask what you would do for a friend or comrade. The patient requires a higher obligation, one that forms out of compassion and trust of the professional for the one asking for his or her special help.

3. *The value of the individual is common to all living bodies.*

   Ethical axiom—Do no harm extends to classes of people, not just to individuals. So, for example, even nontherapeutic medical research carries with it the obligation to do no harm. But the altruism of both the patient and the health care professional, "grounded in the common human condition, can determine that the benefit of no harm can apply to class-instance rather than to the uniqueness of the individual living body." Thus the decision of a physician to ask a terminally ill patient to participate in the testing of a medication that may have dangerous side effects, but will, in the long run benefit those who will come after, is justified as long as the patient agrees.

Traditional biomedical ethicists maintain that ethical dilemmas or conflicting value laden decisions are best made utilizing a form of rational, discursive analysis whose ultimate power is to appeal to objective, rational systems, diminishing any subjectivity, emotion or intuition in order to remain consistent and nonarbitrary. The task becomes one of applying the most appropriate and relevant rule and principle to each situation. Pellegrino and Thomasma[7] have suggested an alternative set of rules that grow out of the unique obligations of health care, and suggest that those rules be considered to be overarching in the decision making process.

Non-Discursive Approach to Ethical Dilemma Resolution

"While acknowledging the power of such rational systems, non-discursive ethicists, however, challenge the narrowness of a strictly applied, formal system of ethical reasoning."[8,p.69] Non-discursive ethicists do *not* claim that discursive ethics is too theoretical or difficult to carry out. Rather their complaint is that theories, principles and rules *alone* promote a formalized, purely objective, cognitive way of thinking that is excessively rational and unbalanced. Too often principles are in conflict. Non-discursive ethicists attempt to balance the process of dilemma resolution by incorporating such aspects of thought as imagination, virtue, character, role, power, discernment and liberation in their search for an adequate method to decide the highest moral alternative.[8]

The Importance of a Person's Story

The final ethical choice, even the decision of which theory seems more compelling, ends versus means, derives from within a personal moral narrative, developed over time, that we all inherit. Robert Nash believes that to restrict ethical decisions to rules and principles alone "sends out the false message that a person's story is irrelevant to (or worse, destructive of) the 'proper' formation of a moral self."[8,p.70] A person's story is a "moral necessity because it provides one with the ethical skills to form one's life truthfully, committedly, and courageously. . .Objective discursive systems allow for rational, step-by-step deliberation and decision making. But the individual's moral intentions and motives originate in, and are formed by, significant people and events in the individual's life."[8,p.70]

The key perspective in discussing the non-discursive aspect of dilemma resolution is to make clear that a choice of the highest moral alternative can be seen to be seated in a rather consistent system of values that can be uncovered by probing one's moral convictions in a deliberate fashion, or by writing a personal ethical autobiography. Once this story is better understood, important questions of character and virtue (What kind of a person am I? and What kind of a person should I be as a health professional?) can be brought up to the light of day. Health professionals must be helped to recognize the way they've set their lenses so that they can adjust to a more professional perspective. For example, if what emerges on self-examination is a preoccupation with self-interest or a fear-laden perspective that takes precedence over autonomy, non-maleficence or beneficence, which are critical to professional health care value decisions, then the health professional must realize that decisions he or she makes very often will not be with highest concern for the welfare of the patient.

Deontology and teleology both presume personal integrity. Principled ethicists believe that one develops moral character and integrity by making rule based decisions justified by ethical principles. Non-discursive ethicists insist that moral character and integrity consist of more than this. To be moral requires constant training as a child and young person, and that training is more than applied ethics. "Integrity is the life-long outcome of actions that shape particular kinds of character. . .And the character that develops is like the narrative of a good novel: it gives a coherence to ethical decisions, and forces individuals to claim their actions as their own."[8,p.71]

As we learned in the previous chapter, cognitive developmental psychologists such as Kohlberg favor a type of training to be moral.[9] They maintain that children are only able to learn how to make higher or more adequate ethical decisions as they develop their cognitive reasoning skills. Moral developmentalists advocate teaching children how to reason morally by teaching them how to solve moral problems. The best moral decisions, according to Kohlberg, are those that are logically consistent and admit to fewer exceptions, respect the dignity of all persons and aim toward just treatment of all people regardless of the law, or of the person's race, creed, color, gender or sexual orientation. Finally, cognitive developmentalists such as Kohlberg and James Rest offer a method of testing that developmental level of moral consciousness of a person by asking them to comment on the moral aspects of a dilemma that they identify as being most relevant. In this way subjects reveal whether they have progressed in their reasoning to an understanding of moral principles or if they remain "stuck" in simply obeying the law or doing that which is socially appropriate.[10]

The Development of Integrity or Consistent Moral Behavior

What kind of a person should I be? Integrity is built from a continuum of choices, some important enough to be remembered, some almost habitual and unreflective. Each time a student cheats in class, or a citizen cheats on reporting income for tax purposes, that choice to behave unethically, no matter what the rationale, wears away at the development of integrity. Choice is not only about what to do in a given situation, choice in making moral decisions is about *who I want to become.* The key question in self-examination is this, "How does a truthful examination of my moral actions fit my moral image of myself?" Do I claim to be a person of virtue and integrity, but choose to participate in gossip, judge others with prejudice, lose my temper, break my promises if I believe they're stupid promises, hurt people under the guise of trying to "help" by being honest, lie when it is expedient to my goals? Answering truthfully requires our lenses to be set to listen carefully to the essential self; the ego must be still. For the ego, the pragmatic goal seeker, will act to get ahead and rationalize that action so that it sounds acceptable, even clever.

How does this detrimental pattern of choice make sense? It makes sense if, in my autobiography I remember the moral axioms of a parent who repeated such phrases to me as, "Get them before they get you." "If you don't look out for yourself, no one else will." "People get what they deserve." "The only thing that matters is who wins." "The winner is the one with the largest or most possessions or salary." "Life is hell and then you die and they throw dirt in your face." This pattern of negative choices also makes more sense today in light of commonly reported ethical lapses by our national and state elected and appointed leaders who most often publicly claim to be highly moral. The moral dictum of "do and say whatever you think will get you re-elected" is the behavior we read about continually. Our country seems to have slipped into a period of the morality of personal gain and expediency. Only now are we waking up to the fact that one result is that we are destroying the planet we live on in the name of personal gain and technological "progress."

Fear-based axioms such as "get them before they get you" are often behind this behavior, and, over time and with repeated exposure, this negativity will seat itself in one's conscience. Feelings of guilt and shame will then surface when you feel someone is out ahead of you, or is better than you are in a class, or when you feel as if you've acted naively or allowed yourself to be taken advantage of.

In a conflict over altruism or beneficence versus self interest or personal gain, it will be difficult to act for the good of your patient when to do so makes you feel as if you've been taken advantage of. Very often day to day ethical decisions are made by deferring to policies and procedures as a way to assuage guilt. For example, a day to day decision of what to do about a walker, paid for by the patient but left behind after her discharge to a nursing home, may not be seen as an ethical decision if one refuses to deal with this mistake because she's "too busy with more important things."

"It's just too bad that the walker was left behind. Thanks for the donation to the department. I don't have time to chase down discharged patients. They're not our concern once they've left this facility." This treatment of a decision ignores the ethical aspect entirely. Selfish concern over the value of one's time versus concern over returning property to its rightful owner and then "passing the buck" by claiming that it's not your fault or problem are attempts to brush away the inadequacy of this mistaken choice.

Thus one's character, built up over the years by listening to important moral statements and making little decisions day after day, will dictate even whether a clinical decision has a moral component to it or not. If a value laden decision is not even recognized, the process of solving the dilemma for the highest good will never even begin.

In other words, being moral means, 1) being able to identify the moral aspect of a problem as well as 2) being a certain kind of person who wants to be able to reason adequately and finally, 3) doing the right thing. Virtue ethicists claim that virtues such as compassion, generosity, fidelity, graciousness, justice and prudence, should be cultivated in people so that doing the right thing becomes consistent with one's character.[11] A person will choose one's ethical behaviors more wisely if they choose in accordance with commonly held virtues. Virtue ethicists argue about which are the most important virtues, of course. Karen Lebaqcz argues that the virtues of fidelity and prudence should be central to the professions. Fidelity to clients includes trustworthiness, promise keeping, honesty and confidentiality; prudence has to do with "an accurate and deliberate perception which enables professionals to perceive realistically what is required in any situation."[12]

Discernment as a Virtue

The common criticism of virtue theory is that cultivating virtue in one's being does not dictate that one will act virtuously in all instances. One might argue that a virtuous person, by definition, would tend to act in a virtuous way, but character traits alone are not enough to ensure the highest moral action.[13]

But if one has reflected on one's values, has paid attention to moral choices, has developed integrity and compassion over time, it becomes easier to act with moral consistency, and inconsistencies serve to stir one's conscience in a way not as available to the morally unaware.

The concept of discernment is integral to the development of character in that discernment is that ability to assert that there is more than objective rationality to moral decision making. Thus, by introducing the whole topic of non-discursive aspects of moral dilemma resolution in this chapter, I am acting on the quality within me of discernment. I believe that the best truth to be found is found within the human decision maker, within the essential self, and every moral decision is a decision that should combine the best of logic and rational methods with attention to the various impulses and movements that occur within a deliberative consciousness.[8]

What is required in day to day ethics is a balance of heart and head, founded in a virtuous moral character that places the good of our patients foremost. Ethical decision making should *never* be reduced to subjectivity and feelings or intuition alone. The non-discursive aspects of moral decision making are not meant to replace the discursive, but to add to it to approach a balance with head and heart. Attention to the non-discursive elements in a moral decision helps one to gain a personal understanding of the moral life. It is in paying attention to this aspect of moral reasoning that one can decide, for example, "when one is willing to make or break a promise, when to tell only the truth, to decide what one is willing to die for."[8,p.75] And to learn to live the consistent and good moral life is one reason why, I believe, we are all here on this earth.

Solving the Ethical Dilemma—A Suggested Process

Ethical dilemmas occur when two or more ethical principles conflict with each other in a given situation and it is unclear what the best or highest moral action would be. Several processes for dilemma resolution have been suggested in the literature.[1-3,6-8,11,12,14] I suggest the following problem solving method be applied to solving ethical dilemmas. It incorporates rule based method with consideration of the consequences and attends to non-discursive elements, as well. This method is an adaptation of the work of Seedhouse and Lovett.[14,pp.19-27]

1. Gather all the *facts* that can be known about this situation.
2. Decide which ethical *principles* are involved—eg, beneficence, nonmaleficence, justice, veracity, autonomy, confidentiality.
3. Clarify your professional *duties* in this situation—eg, do no harm, tell the truth, keep promises, be faithful to colleagues, etc. Duties such as these are often outlined in one's Code of Ethics.
4. Describe the general *nature of the outcome desired,* or the consequences. Which seems most important in this case, an outcome which is most beneficial for the patient, for society, for a particular group or for oneself?
5. Describe pertinent *practical features* of this situation— one or more of the following: disputed facts, the law, the wishes of others, resources available, effectiveness and efficiency of action, the risk, your Code of Ethics and

Standards of Practice, the degree of certainty of the facts on which you base your decision, the predominant values of the others involved (which may or may not coincide with the values predominant in health care in the United States).

When all of the pertinent aspects that go into this particular decision are laid out before you, then you must use your discernment to decide which action is the highest moral alternative. You should be able to justify your decision by explaining both your ethical reasoning process and your conscious weighing of one value over another in this situation, based on what you know about your moral character, the virtues, traditions and beliefs that frame your choices in life, and your professional ethical mandates.

Application of the Suggested Problem Solving Process

Let me illustrate how I would use this process to solve a dilemma. One rather common ethical problem that occurs in spinal cord rehabilitation facilities is the ethical dilemma of what to do when a mentally competent patient refuses beneficial treatment.

Alex is a 23-year-old patient with a cervical fracture and spinal cord lesion at the level of C6-7. He has had a surgical fusion, and he is medically stable and ready to begin rehabilitation, but he refuses to allow others to transfer him from bed to begin the process of tolerating sitting. Testing has revealed normal intelligence and a suspected level of grief and depression following this accident. No active motion has yet been seen below the level of the lesion. The nurses have had problems with his refusal to eat, the physical and occupational therapists have been unable to get him out of bed, the social worker has been unable to engage him in discussion about his depression. He lies in bed with the covers over his head and says, "Leave me alone, I want to die." The physician on the case refuses to take Alex's desires seriously, but also shows little compassion or sensitivity, and commands the orderly to bodily remove Alex from the bed and wheel him to physical therapy. The other members of the team, while not wanting simply to yield indefinitely to Alex's depression, believe that the physician's order is inappropriate and are struggling with what to do. They feel a strong pull of loyalty to other members of the team, including the physician, but resist the "command" to force Alex to comply. They feel a loyalty to their patient, but believe his depression blocks him from making the best decisions for himself at this time.

Application of the Problem Solving Method

1. Gather all of the facts.
   a. Cervical lesion, complete, at C6-7
   b. Young man, 23, no committed relationship to a

    partner, family—father, mother, sister—supporting and visit regularly.

    c. Completed two years of college. Proven intelligence. Taking a year off to "find himself." Risk taker. Athlete.

    d. Accident occurred showing off by diving into shallow water of friend's pool at a party later at night.

    e. From family history, suspected addiction to alcohol, history of risk-taking behaviors.

    f. Family has excellent health insurance.

    g. Friendly, bright personality; strong previous desire to contribute to society. Active in "Big Brothers," Boy Scouts.

    h. Without conferring with the team, the physician has ordered that they act in a way that seems to many to be abusive and insensitive to the patient's hopefully temporary feelings of depression and hopelessness.

2. Decide which ethical principles are involved.

Decision of allowing the patient to have his freedom to act in his own interest, *autonomy,* versus acting in a way to convince the patient to get motivated to begin rehabilitation—*beneficence*—contributing to the overall benefit of the patient. But the other factor is, what is the action that is most beneficial? The doctor's demand to bodily force the patient to comply with a rehab plan may be the end desired, but the means does not seem to be justified. *Above all do no harm* is an issue and a logical question would be, what harm might result from physically forcing the patient to comply? *Fidelity* to one's professional colleague seems to be less important than *do no harm*.

3. Clarify your duties in the situation.

If I am the physical therapist I have a different specific duty than if I am the social worker, occupational therapist, recreation therapist or nurse. But *each* of us has the duty to act in such a way that the patient is supported in overcoming his natural depression and becoming invested in hope for a new life. Once Alex gets beyond his depression and understands at the deepest levels what his choices will be living with quadriplegia, then his decision to live or die will be his to make, free of interference. Right now he doesn't have all of the facts, and his depression keeps him from even considering what those facts might be and how important they are to his decision. In other words, his depression renders him mentally incapable of deciding adequately in his own best interest. My duty as a health professional is to contribute to the team's individual and collective effort to support Alex through his depression, and to help him learn what he can expect from life living with quadriplegia.

I am also obliged to be faithful to my colleagues so that we are united in our approach and work together for a good outcome, but I cannot be faithful to a plan that might cause the patient harm. The physician's order is not one that I can readily follow, so the desire to do no harm and the patient's beneficence seem more important than fidelity to my colleague, the physician.

4. Describe the general nature of the outcome desired.

I want Alex to become involved in rehabilitation and to learn what it is like to be as independent as possible with his quadriplegia, without having to go through the humiliation of being bodily forced to participate in rehabilitation.

5. Describe pertinent practical features of the situation.

disputed facts—1) it is permissible to insist that patients not yield to depression by bodily forcing them to go to rehab. The end justifies the means. This fact can be disputed, as well as, 2) Alex is taking up someone else's bed who wants to be involved in rehab, and someone else "deserves" the rehab bed more.

wishes of others—1) family wants everything done for Alex, as soon as possible. 2) Mother has little tolerance for son's depression. Concurs with physician's order. Father asks for patience and perseverance, plus treatment of depression.

resources available—rehab beds are in demand, but money is not an issue for the family.

risk—forcing Alex to be involved in rehab could cause injury to body or emotions. Also, it may backfire causing more resistance.

degree of certainty of facts—the most uncertain of the facts concerns the nature of the cervical lesion—what will Alex's physical and emotional deficit look like in 6 months, in a year? How debilitated will Alex be, and how independent can we hope he can become? How successful will he be in reforming his core self worth and values so that he might live a fulfilled life as a patient with a disability? Likewise, we are uncertain just how long Alex's depression will last. But even with the uncertainty of the future, the fact *now* is that he is physically ready to participate in rehab. Also certain is the fact that rehab cannot take place successfully without Alex's cooperation. Decision:

1) Meet with the team physician to discuss unwillingness to carry out the order to force Alex to go to rehab.

2) confer with the psychologist, physician, nurse and/or social worker and agree on a plan to systematically confront Alex's depression in a supportive way, with the goal of helping him through it in as timely a way as possible. Commit as a team to giving him the time he needs.

3) once rehab has begun, practice beneficence and "guarded" paternalism while Alex is gaining a sense of himself with his new identity, and then be careful to relinquish any paternalism as Alex becomes able to cognitively and emotionally make decisions for himself, even if the health care team and/or family disagree with those decisions.

Conclusion

Two things seem obvious at this point. Moral decision making takes time, and I may not have considered aspects of this situation that seem quite apparent to you. What if the physician becomes enraged that the team has not followed his instructions and threatens to have each one fired? Sometimes moral stances come to this level of confrontation, but not often. When one's integrity is challenged, it helps to have systematically thought through your decision. I hope you would see that the systematic process itself works to raise the decision making process up out of the murky waters of intuition and subjectivity alone, and I could defend this decision as the best, or highest decision I could make at this time with the facts that I have been given. To go back on this decision because of a threat would weaken my integrity. I would hope that the situation would not come to that end, but if it did, I would be confident in my discernment and would, I hope, remain committed to my decision.

The exercises that follow will first give you a chance to discover more clearly the qualities of your discernment by asking you to write your moral autobiography, and will give you the opportunity to practice ethical dilemma resolution using the suggested process. Remember, you've been making personal moral decisions all of your life. Now what is asked of you is to search for the values, beliefs, stories, myths and parables which have informed those choices in a consistent way. And how well will that way serve you now as a health professional? What changes must you make, if any, to remain true to a commitment to therapeutic presence and healing? Don't forget to journal about your discoveries.

References

1. Purtilo, RB, Cassel, C: *Ethical Dimensions in the Health Professions.* Philadelphia, WB Saunders, 1981.
2. Brody, H: *Ethical Decisions in Medicine.* Boston, Little Brown and Co., 1981.
3. Cahlahan, S: The role of emotion in ethical decision-making. *Hastings Center Report,* June/July, 1988, 9.
4. Kane, RA, Caplan, AL: *Everyday Ethics—Resolving Dilemmas in Nursing Home Life.* New York, Springer Publishing Co., 1990.
5. Guccione, AA: Ethical issues in physical therapy practice. *Phys Ther* 60(10):1264-1272, Oct. 1980.
6. Francoeur, RT: *Biomedical Ethics—A Guide to Decision-Making.* New York, John Wiley and Sons, 1983.
7. Pellegrino, ED, Thomasma, DC: *A Philosophical Basis of Medical Practice.* New York, Oxford University Press, 1981.
8. Nash, RJ: Applied ethics and moral imagination: Issues for educators. *Journal of Thought,* Fall, 1987, pp. 68-77.
9. Kohlberg, L: The cognitive development approach to moral education. *Phi Delta Kappa,* June 1975, pp. 670-677.
10. Munsey, B: *Moral Development, Moral Education and Kohlberg.* Birmingham, Religious Education Press, 1980.
11. Pence, GE: *Ethical Options in Medicine.* Oradell, New Jersey, Medical Economics Company, 1980.
12. Lebaqcz, K: *Professional Ethics: Power and Paradox.* Nashville, Abingdon Press, 1985, pp. 87-99.
13. Purtilo, RB: *Health Professional and Patient Interaction.* 4th ed. Philadelphia, WB Saunders, 1990.
14. Seedhouse, D, Lovett, L: *Practical Medical Ethics.* New York, John Wiley and Sons, 1992.

exercises

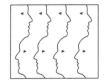

1. Write Your Moral Autobiography

Think back to when you were a child. You may want to interview parents and grandparents for more information.

What do you remember being punished for? What were your siblings punished for?

What were the rules of the family? Where did those rules seem to come from? The Bible? The church? From ancient wisdom passed down?

What were you praised for? What were you encouraged to do?

Were there certain favorite virtues that were emphasized?

What were the family rules for making decisions, or did that remain a mystery?

What was your favorite fairy tale or myth? What is the moral lesson to that story? Have you incorporated it into your actions?

What do you remember being most emotional about? Did you have a favorite cause? Have you ever participated in a march for a cause or in any actions of civil disobedience? Would you, if you were challenged to? Why or why not?

Recount any major moral decisions you remember making, any moral stands you have taken. Write a story of the development of your moral consciousness.

2. Examine Your Code of Ethics

Locate a copy of your profession's Code of Ethics. Analyze the Code statements to determine the values and ethical principles that are most esteemed by your profession. Next examine the Code for what it seems to be missing. What would you wish the Code would speak to, but doesn't?

3. Values Discovery

List the values you believe are the prominent values in *society* today (for example, freedom of speech). Then list the values which were prominent in your *family* (for example, go to church on Saturday or Sunday). List the values you hold dear as an *individual* (for example, love your neighbor).

Next list the values you found to be most important in your profession (eg, above all, do no harm). List the values you have observed in an area where patients are being treated by fellow professionals (eg, first come, first served). Finally, list what you perceive to be one individual's values as he or she practices your profession with patients (eg, confidentiality).

Compare and contrast each set of values to your individual values. How well do they fit? What values listed can be located in your Code of Ethics? Which values are not contained in your Code?

4. Ethical Dilemma Resolution

Below are several day-to-day dilemmas faced by health professionals. Choose one. Go through the process to resolve it as illustrated in the chapter above. Solve it first from a teleological perspective, then solve it from a principle or deontological perspective. Do you come to the same moral conclusion? Why or why not?

a. A physical therapist colleague in private practice admits that he charges less money for patients who pay with cash because he never records this income for tax purposes. You have been working for this therapist for 6 months, and in order to keep your job, he is asking you to adopt the same system, and offers you a cash bonus of $5,000.00 at Christmas because you deserve the money more than the IRS. Personal circumstances make this the only place where you can practice and still fulfill your family responsibilities. You are the only person in your family employed at the time, and you are supporting two children and an elderly mother.

b. You have agreed to "fill in" for a home care therapist for two weeks. At four of the five patients' homes in one day, as you evaluated and treated according to your standards, the patients have made comments that the other therapist never did any of this kind of therapy. It becomes apparent to you that the therapist you are filling in for is giving no professional care. You are scheduled to move out of this town as soon as this two-week time period ends to another state. If you report this person, you may be required to return to this state at your own expense to testify. Your finances are very meager. School loans and debts result in your living on a tight budget from pay period to pay period. To come back and testify you would have to borrow the money.

c. At 4:45 a woman in severe pain walks into the physical therapy department with a referral from her physician to be evaluated and treated for severe low back pain. The physical therapist in charge (and the only one present) had stayed late to see patients well after the usual closing time of 5:00 for the past week. Further, the day care center had called just before the woman walked in, stating that the therapist's six-month-old daughter was very sick, with severe vomiting and diarrhea, and they were very worried about her. The therapist's wife is out of town. The therapist tells the patient, "I'm sorry, we're closed for the day and I *must* leave. You'll have to come back in the morning." The woman bursts into tears and says she doesn't even know if she can make it home, she is in such pain.

section two

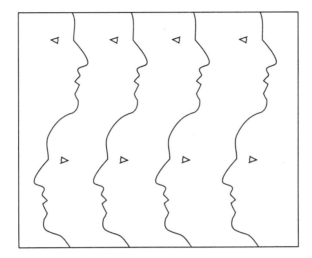

INTERACTING WITH OTHERS

This second section is composed of six chapters devoted to examining ways in which we interact with our patients and our colleagues. Chapter Five introduces this topic with an examination of the nature of effective helping—what makes help helpful? If you've ever felt victimized by a well meaning person who insists on helping you when you don't want to be helped, you've experienced help that is not helpful. The characteristics of helpful help and the characteristics of effective helpers are both examined. The concepts of compassion and empathy are explored in relation to effective help. Empathy is distinguished from its similar interactional processes such as sympathy, pity, identification, association and self transposal. This chapter concludes with a closer look at the values that are conducive to helpful help, thus conducive to healing.

Chapter Six introduces the development of a package of skills: problem identification, active listening and "I" statements. Use of these techniques establishes a way of communicating effectively in the helper-helpee relationship. These skills also will assist you as you learn to be assertive in the face of tension. Chapter Seven presents assertiveness skill development and Chapter Eight teaches you how to conduct a patient interview.

Section Two continues with Chapter Nine in which we examine the particular characteristics of effective interaction with those who are dying. Death is, for most of us, an uneasy reality that we would rather not have to consider as a natural part of our lives on earth. Depending on our profession and specialty, many of us will be called upon to care for those who have a limited time left on earth. It is helpful to have considered in advance the actions that are most caring and healing, and to be aware of potentially hurtful or harmful ways of communicating in these situations. But even more important, considering our own limited time on the earth, we become intensely more aware of our selves, of our priorities, of the attitudes and values that underlie a life of quality. Once you've experienced the readings and activities in Chapter Nine, you should know much more than just how to communicate in a healing manner with the terminally ill. You will know more about your self.

Chapter Ten concludes this section and the text itself. In this chapter we examine the concept of burnout, or the professional exhaustion sometimes experienced by health professionals especially when they are confronted with problems that seem unsolvable or goals that seem unreachable. The final advice this text can offer you is that, when you are communicating well with your patients and colleagues, and taking a regular personal inventory of your feelings and the issues in your life as the journal process of this text has facilitated, burnout will be less likely to occur. For the first step to preventing burnout is recognition of the problem. Nonetheless, emotional stress is, at times, inevitable. The key is to interrupt the process before it escalates. This chapter will help develop habits that will assist you in that process.

Best of luck!

chapter five

THE NATURE OF EFFECTIVE HELPING

Objectives

1. To consider the overall aim of helping.
2. To explore the behaviors that interfere with effective helping.
3. To describe the characteristics of helping communication.
4. To distinguish empathy from related interpersonal interaction processes.
5. To reveal the characteristics of effective helpers.

When someone needs help, no matter what the nature of the help needed, we can assume that something's not right, something is interfering with day-to-day function and growth. Those of us in the healing professions have devoted our lives, for the most part, to helping those who need help in understanding and overcoming illness or disability. Some of us, however, are more concerned with working with people who are, essentially, well but need help in becoming more fit, or need help in preventing illness or injury. Whatever the problem, health professionals have devoted their professional lives to helping people overcome whatever is blocking them from living functionally useful and productive lives.

What should the overall aim of helping be? When we were small and needed help, we searched out whomever we felt could fix the problem and make us feel better. As children, we lacked the skills to solve our own problems, and so we depended on our mothers and fathers, or some capable adult to take charge. Unlike children, adults require a different sort of helping, for when someone constantly tries to "fix it," we often become resentful and angry and feel helpless and dependent. It is an important sign of maturity when we prefer to complete tasks and solve problems ourselves, and take pride in our individual accomplishments.

There are times, however, when we feel particularly alone and helpless and we may appreciate that "fixing" kind of attention and help offered by a friend. Remember the comment from a previous chapter that greeting cards emphasize this common human need in phrases like, "Before I even knew my own needs, you were there with a loving heart to respond." But this sentiment fails to acknowledge the more enduring need for adults to feel self-sufficient and capable of identifying and solving their own problems.

The overall aim of mature helping always is to make the helpee self-sufficient, to assist the helpee in achieving a more effective relationship between self and others and between self and the world.

We have discovered in previous chapters that our behavior is an expression of our values and our beliefs. Those who believe they are called to help others whether they want help or not can become annoying at the least and obstructive to others' development at the worst. Not all help is helpful. Many of us have laughed at the turmoil that can occur when a well-meaning person tries to open a door for us and actually blocks our way. At the other end of the continuum, however, is the well-meaning friend or parent who takes great care in telling us what to do in a given situation, then abandons us with indifference, refusing to support us until we comply with the advice given.

As was pointed out in Chapter Two, helpers who have grown up in troubled homes and thus developed parenting skills too early bring immature ideas about the nature of effective help into adulthood. A few familiar characteristics of "unhelpful helpers" include an overconcern with matters that are none of their business, a need to be told how helpful, indeed, how irreplaceable they are to the functioning of a group, and a need to have others depend on them as if their very self-worth revolved totally around their ability to fix problems for others. And, sadly, often it does.

The important truth in this matter is that no person can take responsibility for another person. We can only take responsibility for ourselves. Exceptions exist, of course, with children and with people who, for whatever reason, have lost the ability to be adequately in charge of their own lives—those with certain mental illnesses, those with brain dysfunction.

Effective helping usually has as a primary component a problem identification and problem solving process. As health professionals, we learn important knowledge, skills and values that we offer to assist those needing help to understand the nature of their problem(s) and to act in ways so that the problem is solved and a return to normal function and quality living is facilitated. Our goal must always be to help the helpee become self-sufficient once again. We must provide the conditions for our patients to identify their own goals around their health problem, and provide the knowledge and skill to advise them on the wisdom of their desires, and then to help them get their needs met.

Patients may come to us with or without a diagnosis, but, contrary to common practice in most medical environments, the diagnosis serves as little more than a place to start in the helping process. The key questions remain: What are the problems from the patient's perspective? And what are the patient's goals in the healing process? Effective helping includes not merely a provision of information and therapeutic procedures, but involves helping the patient with the discovery of personal meaning as well.

Therapeutic Use of Self

Central to this perspective on helping is therapeutic communication, and the therapeutic use of one's self. How you view yourself will markedly affect your communication. Remember that the self-concept acts as a screen through which we view the world. Most of us have felt the discomfort of interacting with a person who continually apologizes for him or herself, who distorts what we say out of feelings of insecurity, who responds with negativity and self-contempt. Each of us holds many varied opinions and ideas about ourselves, but our essential self-worth forms the core around which those ideas merge, and negative self-worth is one of the most important factors that needs to be changed in order to communicate from a healing perspective. Section One of this text focuses on the development of the ideas about the self, and how our feelings of self-worth evolve. This chapter focuses on the nature of effective communication in the helping process.

Therapeutic Communication

Certain identifiable elements characterize therapeutic or healing communication. In the practitioner-patient interaction, the practitioner:

- Speaks—Communicates not just with an expression of ideas but with the ability to translate those ideas from an inner conviction to an outer clarity. Self-awareness enables the speaker to voice articulately well-thought-out ideas regarding the role of the patient in the healing process.
- Is fully present—Is totally focused on the patient and his or her ideas about the problem. Does not get lost in memories of "patients past" or possible future problems. Allows the interaction with the patient to command his or her full attention.
- Listens—Listens with the whole self, with the "third ear" in order to ascertain the patient's meanings and goals. Clarifies interpretations of what is heard. Resists categorizing or projecting personal beliefs and values. Resists giving quick advice, telling the patient what to do.
- Develops trust—Resists trying to influence the patient; instead, asks questions only to ascertain the truth about the problem as the patient perceives it. Communicates that the patient is worth listening to, that he or she has important information to add to this process. Resists assuming a priestly or parental role that conveys that the patient is dumb and that he or she is smart. At the same time, however, conveys the values of expertise and confidentiality, and never neglects the opportunity for

informed consent so that the patient feels that trust has been appropriately placed.

Thus the art of professional helping in the healing professions centers around the therapeutic use of oneself by way of a style of humanistic communication that places the patient in a position of informed equal, inevitably responsible for any positive outcomes in the helping process.

Health professionals:

- listen, clarify, ask, never assume or make quick judgments
- identify problems with the patient, evaluate
- hypothesize causes
- treat through therapeutic measures and education
- reevaluate
- readjust to the new state and begin again until goals are reached

A Closer Look at Interpersonal Interaction

At the heart of listening with the "third ear" is the process of self transposal, which is often confused with empathy.[1] *Empathy* (Figure 5-1) is very often used interchangeably with several other interaction terms. Each term has a unique meaning and it is helpful to understand and be able to distinguish among them. The terms most commonly used interchangeably with empathy include sympathy, pity, identification and self transposal. Of these, pity and identification often are not appropriate to the healing process. Let's take a closer look at each of these interactive processes.

When I *sympathize* (Figure 5-2) with you, I feel similar feelings about something outside of us along with you. I can feel joyful about your success, or I can feel sadness about the bad news that my patient received today. This is sympathy, or "fellow feeling." It is very commonly felt in health care and it is totally appropriate in the healing relationship with patients.

Pity (Figure 5-2), on the other hand, rarely, if ever, is appropriate. When I pity my patient, I feel sympathy with condescension. "You poor thing," conveys an inappropriate inequality between myself and the other person; I lift myself up to be better than the other, and in that process, I demean the personhood of the other. Granted, pity may draw us to help others, but to help with condescension gives the message to the patient that you are judging him or her to be "pitiful."

Identification (Figure 5-2) can interfere with healing communication, as well. When I identify with my patient, I begin to feel at one with him or her and in that process, I often lose sight of the differences between us. For example, just because we both have the same last name, or we both come from similar backgrounds, I may forget that he or she might have different values than I do. I may assume my patient feels as I do about wanting to know everything there is to know about a disease or disorder, or I may project that my patient is at her best in the morning, and schedule her before noon. I forget to ask, to clarify. As a result, I confuse my meanings and values with those of my patient; I project my values onto the patient and act in ways that make the patient less important, less relevant to the healing

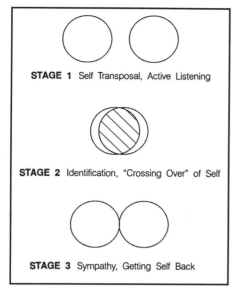

Figure 5-1. Three stages of empathy as described by Stein.

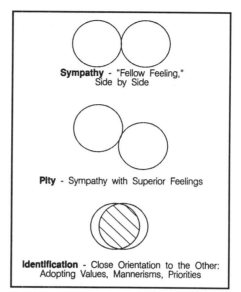

Figure 5-2. Graphic representation of three intersubjective processes.

process. In addition, as I identify, or become one with the patient, I risk losing my own perspective, which weakens my therapeutic objectivity, and I often become very subjective in the information I convey. Identification with patients often leads to an over-friendliness with patients and an inappropriate sharing of personal information that can interfere with the therapeutic nature of the relationship. I'll expand on this more before the end of this chapter.

Self transposal is a cognitive "thinking of myself" into the position of the other. It is the process most often confused with empathy, putting myself in the other's place, or more commonly, walking a mile in another person's shoes. In his earlier writings, Carl Rogers refers to this as empathy, but in truth, self transposal merely sets the stage for empathy to occur. In self transposal, I listen carefully and try to imagine what it must be like for the patient to be experiencing what he or she is describing.

The process of empathy was first fully described by Edith Stein.[2] In her scholarly work, published in the 1930s, Stein characterizes empathy as absolutely unique from all other forms of interactions, distinguishable from other intersubjective processes first by the fact that we never empathize; empathy happens to us. It "catches" us. It is given to us much like true forgiveness; when it finally comes, it seems to be given to us. We can want to forgive, and try to forgive, but when the forgiveness finally comes, there is a sense in which we haven't done a thing except allowed it to come.

Second, empathy takes place in three overlapping stages. The first stage is the cognitive attending to the other, or self transposal, as described above. We listen carefully in an attempt to put ourselves in the place of the other. The second stage, following just a millisecond after, is, by far, the most significant. This is the "crossing over" stage, wherein we feel our selves crossing over for a moment into the frame of reference, or the lived world of the other person. We feel so at one with the other, we forget momentarily that we are two separate beings. This is the identification stage of empathy.

The third stage resolves the temporary confusion, as we come back into our "own skin," and feel a special alignment with the other after having experienced the crossing over. This third stage resembles sympathy, or "fellow feeling." Thus empathy can be described as a momentary merging with another person in a unique moment of shared meaning. Elsewhere I describe this process in more depth as it occurs within physical therapists for their patients.[1]

When empathy occurs, helping professionals need not lose their therapeutic objectivity, as so many fear, in getting "too close" to their patients. Instead what is experienced is a kind of holistic listening that can unite the therapist with the patient, yet allows the patient and therapist to remain fully separate in the healing process. It is in identification alone that we lose our objectivity and become destructively fused with the patient, as described earlier.

Thus, empathy is the intersubjective process that, among other things, empowers us to listen with the "third ear," to communicate humanistically and therapeutically with patients, thus contributing to helpful helping.

Levels of Intimacy in Professional Interaction

The challenge, then, is for the health professional to be in therapeutic relationship with patients, yet maintain the helper-helpee relationship. It is imperative that this relationship remain functional, always serving the purpose of healing. How does the clinician reveal just enough about herself or himself to maintain the trust and collegiality without allowing the relationship to change into a more involved friendship or intimate relationship? Revealing too much might confuse the patient by seeming to convey that you are willing to give more than is appropriate for the helping process. Powell[3] describes five different levels of communication that one can use as guidelines for communicating effectively without revealing too much about oneself. These levels lie on a continuum from near indifference to extreme intimacy.

- Level Five: Cliche Conversation
  No genuine human sharing takes place. "How are you?" "It's nice to see you." Protects people from each other and prevents the likelihood of meaningful communication.
- Level Four: Reporting Facts
  Almost nothing personal is revealed. Some sharing takes place about information such as diagnostic data or the weather.
- Level Three: Personal Ideas and Judgments
  Some information about oneself is shared, often in response to the patient's conversation. Topics talked about often relate to the patient's

illness or the process the patient is going through, and if the patient looks bored or confused, conversation reverts back to level four.

- Level Two: Feelings and Emotions
  A deep trust is required to share at this level, and if a person fears judgment, it will be impossible to relate at this level. True friendship and caring require this level of communication. Each person wants to be deeply known and accepted just as he or she is.

- Level One: Peak Communication
  Mutual complete openness, honesty, respect and love are required to communicate at this level. An all-encompassing intimacy is shared, often involving relating sexually. The minority of human interactions take place at this level.

In therapeutic communication with patients, it is important for the professional to have a clear idea about appropriate boundaries that will facilitate healing. Once crossed over, interaction beyond this boundary will confuse patients, and the health professional will appear to be offering more of him or herself to the relationship than is facilitative to the helper-helpee relationship.

In most instances, interaction will take place at levels five, four and three with an occasional interchange at level two, but never at level one.

New professionals often confuse the appropriate boundaries and find themselves caring too much, spending more time with one patient than is wise, or telling inappropriate stories or jokes in an attempt to make the patient feel at ease. The reverse often occurs when the patient feels compelled to help put the practitioner at ease. Patients don't need this added anxiety; they need to relax and trust that the health professional has his or her best interests at heart, and can manage the healing interaction free of awkwardness or threats to confidentiality and trust.

Beliefs of Effective Helpers

A.W. Combs[4] and colleagues at the University of Florida have conducted research on the characteristics of effective helpers and concluded, "Good helpers are not born, nor are they made in the sense of being taught. . .Becoming a helper is a time-consuming process. It is not simply a matter of learning methods or of acquiring gadgets and gimmicks. It is a deeply personal process of exploration and discovery, the growth of unique individuals learning over a period of time how to use themselves effectively for helping other people."

Helpers were evaluated for their effectiveness, and the most effective responded to specific questions about their beliefs in six major categories. The results are summarized in Table 5-1.

These beliefs are all developed in a growth process that is very much influenced by the way the lenses we talked about in earlier chapters are set. The key to becoming an effective helper is to allow one's self to grow, to mature, to become more aware of feelings as well as thoughts, to be able to

Table 5-1.
Summary of the Beliefs of "Effective" Helpers

Combs, et al. describe commonly held beliefs and perceptions of effective helpers in six categories:

1. **Subject or Discipline**
   One is committed to knowing one's discipline well, but mere knowledge is not enough. Knowledge about one's discipline is so personally integrated and meaningful as to have the quality of belief. Effective helpers are committed to discovering the personal meaning of knowledge and converting it to belief.

2. **Helper's Frame of Reference**
   Effective helpers tend to favor an internal frame of reference emphasizing the importance of people's attitudes, feelings and values that are uniquely human over an external frame of reference that emphasizes facts, things, organization, money, etc.

3. **Beliefs About People**
   Effective helpers believe that people are essentially:
   • able to understand and deal with their own problems given sufficient time and information.
   • basically friendly and well-intentioned
   • worthy and have great value; they possess dignity and integrity which must be maintained.
   • essentially internally motivated, maturing from within and striving to grow and help themselves.
   • a source of satisfaction in professional work rather than a source of suspicion and frustration.

4. **Helper's Self-Concept**
   Effective helpers have a clear sense of self and their own personal boundaries before they enter into relationships with others. They feel basically fulfilled and adequate, so self-discipline is well practiced. Therapeutic presence for the other is made possible by a strong sense of self, of personal fulfillment and of personal adequacy.

5. **Helper's Purposes**
   Effective helpers believe that their purpose is to facilitate and assist rather than control people. They favor responding to the larger issues, the broader perspective rather than the minute details in life. They tend to be willing to be themselves, to be self-revealing. Their purpose includes honesty, acknowledging personal inadequacies and need for growth. Another purpose is to be involved and committed to the helping process. They are process oriented and committed to working out solutions rather than working toward preconceived goals or notions. They see themselves as altruistic, oriented toward assisting people rather than simply responding to selfish needs.

6. **Beliefs About Appropriate Methods or Approaches to the Task**
   Effective helpers are more oriented toward people than toward rules and regulations or things. They are more concerned about people's perceptions than with the objective framework within which they practice. In helping people, the most effective approach is to discover how the world seems to that person. Self-concept is at the heart of the way one views the world, and so working with self-concept is imperative. Helpers have to be committed to gaining the trust of helpees so that self-control can be relearned in a positive way. The helping relationship makes this growth possible.

Combs, AW: *Florida Studies in the Helping Professions.* Gainesville, FL, University of Florida Press, 1969.

identify those beliefs that lead to behaviors that facilitate healing, and grow beyond defensive behaviors that result in negativity and fragmentation.

Professionals will act according to what they believe their purpose is. The purpose of the mature healing professional is to listen carefully, with the "third ear"; to evaluate; to assist; to support; to help problem solve alternatives that lead to healing; to apply therapeutic measures aimed at alleviating pain and dysfunction; to teach; to help others discover how to maneuver successfully in the world and to solve their own problems that interfere with the highest and deepest functioning possible.

Carl Rogers[5] suggests seven key questions that lead to a form of self-examination that will help us evaluate the quality of one's helping:

1. Can I behave in some way which will be perceived by the other person as trustworthy, as dependable or consistent in some deep sense?

   Here congruence is the key factor. Whatever feeling or attitude is being experienced must be matched by an awareness of that attitude and actions must match feelings.

2. Can I be expressive enough as a person that what I am will be communicated unambiguously?

   The difficulty here is to be fully aware of who one truly is. Rogers says this: ". . .if I can form a helping relationship to myself—if I can be sensitively aware of and acceptant toward my own feelings—then the likelihood is great that I can form a helping relationship toward another."

3. Can I let myself experience positive attitudes toward this other person—attitudes of warmth, caring, liking, interest, respect?

   This often engenders the fear that if we allow ourselves to openly express these feelings, the helpee might misinterpret our intentions, and the therapeutic distance might be blurred. The key here is to remain in our professional identities and yet still relate in a caring way to the other person.

4. Can I be strong enough as a person to be separate from the other?

   This question speaks to avoiding identification. I must be ever aware of my own feelings and express them as mine, totally separate from the feelings I may perceive that the helpee is experiencing. Likewise, I must be strong in my otherness to avoid becoming depressed when my patient is depressed, or fearful in the face of my patient's fear, or destroyed by his or her anger.

5. Can I let myself enter fully into the world of [my patient's] feelings and personal meanings and see these as [he or she] does?

   The key effort here is to avoid judging the patient's perspectives, but instead allow empathy to occur. In this way, once the world of the other is more fully experienced, the help that is offered can be based on this holistic level of knowing made possible by empathy. Meanings can be confronted with acceptance and modified to work toward healing. Judgment and criticism of meanings places a barrier between the helper and the helpee.

6. Can I act with sufficient sensitivity in the relationship that my behavior will not be perceived as a threat?

A patient who feels free of external fear or threat feels free to examine behavior and change it. Patient care is threatening in and of itself. Whatever we can do to lower anxiety will assist the effectiveness of our helping.

7. Can I meet this other individual as a person who is in the process of becoming, or will I be bound by his [or her] past and by my past?

Martin Buber uses the phrase "confirming the other." This means accepting the whole potentiality of the other,. . .the person he [or she] was created to become.[6] People will act the way we relate to them. The Pygmalion effect was described following the famous Broadway play in which a poor working girl showed that she could behave like a princess when she was treated like one and taught carefully.

The more one fully comprehends the importance of the nature of the helping interaction, the more one will become committed to the growth required for consistent therapeutic use of self. Yes, our professional knowledge and skill are critical to our effectiveness, but without the ability to interact in healing ways, we sabotage most efforts.

Awareness Through Action

The exercises that follow are aimed at helping you discover your currently held ideas about the nature of helping, and why you are interested in becoming a health professional. Your beliefs about your self are explored, and you are given the opportunity to practice one of the major factors of effective helping: active listening. You'll be surprised how difficult it is to really hear what someone else is saying.

References

1. Davis, CM: *A Phenomenological Description of Empathy as it Occurs Within Physical Therapists for their Patients.* Unpublished doctoral dissertation. Boston, Boston University, 1982.
2. Stein, E: *On the Problem of Empathy.* Second Ed. The Hague, Martinus Nijhoff, 1970.
3. Powell, J: *Why Am I Afraid to Tell You Who I Am?* Niles, Illinois, Argus Communications, 1969.
4. Combs, AW, Avila, DL, Purkey, WW: *Helping Relationships—Basic Concepts for the Health Professions.* Second edition. Boston, Allyn and Bacon, Inc. 1971.

5. Rogers, C: The characteristics of a helping relationship. In Rogers, C: *On Becoming a Person.* Boston, Houghton, Mifflin, 1961.
6. Buber, M, Rogers, C: Transcription of dialogue held April 18, 1957, Ann Arbor, MI. Unpublished manuscript.
7. Simon, SB, Howe,, L, Kirschenbaum, H: Values clarification—A Handbook for Teachers. New York, Hart Publishers, 1972.

exercises

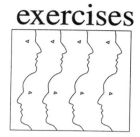

1. Self Awareness/Why Do I Want To Help?

Respond to the following questions. Discuss with two or three others and then with the entire class. Note the variety of reasons why people are drawn to the helping professions, and note the responses most of you share in common.

1. Why do I want to be a helping professional?

2. Whom do I most want to help?

3. What specific rewards do I get from helping people?

4. How do I want to be perceived by those I intend to help?

5. Do I believe people are essentially lazy and will want to have me do all the work for them, or do I believe people most of the time want to help themselves? Is there a category of patients who I believe are mostly lazy? How did I decide this?

6. I feel most anxious when I'm helping, when?

7. Those who require the most help from others are, who?

8. Answering these questions made me feel, what?

Journal Reflections

As I reflect on my response to the above questions, what did I learn about myself?

2. **Beliefs About Self**

Complete the following self awareness continuum. Discuss with a person in the class that you trust and can be open and honest with. Compare your responses to the beliefs of effective helpers as outlined in Table 5-1.

What I Believe About Myself Today

1. Identification

   Feel apart from those I work with. Important to keep my distance, stay somewhat aloof.

   Identify with others; I feel a part of those I work with, those I lead, those who are my patients.

   X _____ X

2. Adequacy

   Life is very complex and I flounder a lot in trying to keep it together for myself. Hard to keep aware of all my choices in life.

   Most of the time I'm capable of solving my own problems, at least dealing with them. Life situations usually offer several choices for me to make and I usually do okay.

   X _____ X

3. Trust

   The future of my health profession is somewhat shaky. I may not have a job; my curriculum is somewhat tenuous dependent solely on the quality of various instructors that come and go. I may end up not being able to help much.

   Basically, I feel I am a dependable, reliable person, capable of coping with the future of health care and of coping with my new growth no matter where it leads me.

   X _____ X

4. Degree of feeling wanted.

   Most days I feel pretty rejected and ignored. People on the whole don't act like they really want me around.

   I may not be most attractive person in the world, but mostly I feel I am essentially likable, attractive and wanted.

   X _____ X

5. Worthiness

   My worthiness and integrity are often overlooked by most people, especially by those who really matter to me.

   I feel I am a person of consequence, dignity, integrity and worthy respect.

   X _____ X

Adapted from Beliefs of Professional Workers in Combs, AW, Avila, DL, Purkey, WW: *Helping relationships—Basic concepts for the helping professions.* Boston, Allyn and Bacon, 1971.

3. Effective Listening

According to Rogers, good listening involves:

1. Not only hearing the words of the speaker, but hearing the feelings behind the words as well.
2. Putting oneself in the place of the other, or self transposal; feeling the other's feelings and seeing the world through the speaker's eyes.
3. Suspending one's own value judgments so as to understand the speaker's thoughts and feelings as he or she experiences them.

Really listening is very difficult and takes practice, especially if you disagree with what is being said. Most normal conversations involve talking *at* one another rather than *with* one another.

Divide into groups of three. One person serves as monitor, the other two as discussants. The monitor helps the discussants find a topic of mutual interest but one on which they fundamentally disagree. The first discussant states his or her position. In the typical discussion, we are so concerned with what we are going to say next, or so involved with planning our response, that we often tune out or miss the full meaning of what is being said. In this exercise, before any discussant offers a point of view, he or she must first summarize the essence of the previous speaker's statement, so that the previous speaker honestly feels his or her statement has been understood. *It is the monitor's role to see that this process takes place with each exchange.*[7]

Discussion takes place for ten minutes with the monitor assuming the responsibility of insuring that the procedure described above is followed. At the end of ten minutes, discussants give each other feedback about how well they felt they had been heard, understood and responded to.

The process is repeated with the monitor assuming the role of discussant and one of the discussants becoming monitor.

One more note: The role of monitor is critical to the success of this exercise. The monitor *must* insist that each person summarize the other's statement before speaking. This is difficult to do, but essential to the success of the exercise. So, be insistent, and be brave!

chapter six

EFFECTIVE COMMUNICATION
PROBLEM IDENTIFICATION AND HELPFUL RESPONSES

Objectives

1. To teach communication strategies for interactions that are confused and/or emotion laden.
2. To define congruence and give the opportunity to examine one's own congruence or lack of it.
3. To emphasize the importance of both thoughts and feelings in communication.
4. To point out the risks and rewards of communicating clearly in the presence of intense feelings.

Very often the bulk of our communication throughout the day is quite superficial. Rarely do we communicate with the express purpose of trying to understand in order to be helpful. Even when we make a greater than usual attempt to listen carefully because we care and are concerned, it is rare that our interaction might be said to be truly helpful. Therapeutic communication requires learning a new skill, but more than that, it requires unlearning habitual, non-helpful ways of interacting. This chapter is devoted to teaching you a new way of communicating with the express purpose of developing your abilities to use communication as an integral aspect of your therapeutic presence with patients. It might be helpful to begin with a case example.

> Jonathan was enjoying the seventh month of his first position as a physical therapist in a rehabilitation center. Each day he was experiencing more confidence in his skills in evaluation and treatment, especially using therapeutic exercise for patients with spinal cord and brain injury. One of his favorite patients was a young, 14-year-old high school cheerleader who had been referred to him two months ago while still in a coma in the intensive care unit. Diane had gone through the front windshield of her mother's car, a consequence of not having her seatbelt fastened. Her mother escaped injury, but was feeling tremendous guilt. She and Diane had been arguing at the time and she mistakenly ran a stoplight that resulted in the accident.
>
> Just last week Diane began to respond to light and sound, and yesterday she opened her eyes and looked at Jonathan for the first time after he had transferred her to a chair at bedside. He was feeling elated, and was very hopeful that soon she would be responding to verbal commands.
>
> Diane's mother visited every day, and often was present while Jonathan treated Diane. Today Mrs. Graham seemed particularly discouraged. Even though Diane was showing obvious signs of recovery from her coma, she was still unable to move. When Jonathan came to treat Diane, Mrs. Graham left the room, but returned as he finished and told him she wanted to speak to him. As they walked out into the hallway, Mrs. Graham turned to Jonathan and shouted, "You're not helping her! No one is helping her recover. I asked around and found out you're a new therapist and you can't know what you're doing or my daughter would have been well long before this! I want you to stop seeing her. I want a therapist with experience to treat my daughter. I never want you to set foot in her room again!"

The above is an example of an emotion-laden interaction similar to many that take place daily in hospitals and health care facilities. If you were Jonathan, how would you have responded? What would you have felt? Would you have quickly defended yourself? Would you have argued that Diane was showing remarkable signs of improvement? Would you have shouted, "Nobody speaks to me like that!"?

When people are ill and injured, emotions run high both on the part of the ill and their families and on the part of those who are caring for them. Illness and injury stir up feelings of vulnerability and fear. People generally feel out of control, and must give over control of their lives to strangers, often in institutions which seem like strange, impersonal, frightening cultures all their own.

At the root of every emotion-laden interaction is a problem. What, exactly, is the problem in this situation, and whose problem is it? Mrs. Graham would say that the problem is that her daughter is being treated by an inexperienced physical therapist and is not recovering because of it. Therefore, Jonathan and his inexperience are the problem. Jonathan might say that the problem was that Mrs. Graham was feeling helpless and responsible for her daughter's pain and injury, and lashed out at him in her frustration. Another analysis might offer that the problem is that Diane did not have her seatbelt on, and if she had, she would not even be in a coma.

This chapter focuses on identifying problems and clarifying problem ownership in interchanges that are characterized by intense emotions. In the midst of an interchange like the above, it is often difficult to sort out what is happening and what might be appropriate responses that would help resolve the situation. Different skills are required depending on the nature of the problem and who "owns" the problem.

The underling theme in this chapter is this: communicating in ways that help to solve problems, while at the same time respecting and honoring human beings, will facilitate the healing process. Because we work with people who are ill or disabled, it is not enough simply to make the correct diagnosis and give the most appropriate treatment. Something more is expected of us. That "something more" includes helping the patient understand his or her illness or disability to the extent that he or she can make choices with regard to treatment and with regard to modifying lifestyles to prevent further problems and to live successfully with the problems that are not going to be resolved.

Learning New Communication Skills

Each of us enters the helping professions having communicated all of our lives. It doesn't take much patient care experience to learn that the communication skills that served us quite adequately in our private lives often fall short of helping us to relate adequately to patients and colleagues in day-to-day patient care. As Dr. Eric Cassell writes in his book, *Talking with Patients,*[1] without effective communication we are unable to acquire objective and subjective information in order to make decisions that are in the best interests of the patient, and, more importantly, we are unable to utilize the relationship between practitioner and patient for therapeutic ends. This chapter focuses on sorting out emotion-laden communication in order to help patients identify and solve their own problems. Chapter Seven extends this theme in teaching you the skills of assertiveness, and Chapter Eight will instruct you in carrying out a helping interview.

Emotion-Laden Interchanges

Communication connects us to the world. Humans are essentially social, and need to feel a connection to others. Getting our basic needs met more often than not requires some form of communication.

Barriers to the effectiveness of communication might include the use of a foreign language (or the use of jargon), carelessness in choosing the words that convey exact meaning, and/or an inability or unwillingness to listen to each other carefully (hearing deficit, distraction by environmental "noise," unwillingness to concentrate, defensiveness). Many of us are rather unaware of how effective we are in day-to-day communication. It is difficult to come outside of ourselves and watch ourselves interact with others, reflecting on our feelings and the way in which we react to others. Others of us have been given direct feedback about our communication. Statements such as "I love the way you listen so intently to what I say, and wait until I'm finished before you respond." versus "I wish you'd hear me out instead of mentally practicing a quick comeback!" give us clear information about how we're doing as we communicate in that moment.

The fundamentals of communication consist of a sender, a message, a receiver and an environment. In an emotion-laden interchange, the message is obscured by the fact that someone is upset and unable to identify clearly what the heart of the problem is, and how to best go about solving it. What is most important is that you realize that the luxury you experienced as a "private citizen" before you made a commitment to becoming a health professional of simply reacting to others must now be replaced by a commitment to use emotion-laden communication (even when you feel personally attacked), as an opportunity to practice your therapeutic effectiveness.

Less Than Helpful Responses

The most unhelpful response is indifference. To fail to listen is indicative of an inability or unwillingness to be therapeutically present to the one in need of help. Other less than helpful techniques include the following[2]:

- Offering Reassurances
  Statements such as, "Oh, it can't be all that bad" or "If you think you have it bad, you should just look around you" do little but signal an unwillingness to listen to patients' perceptions of their problems. At the heart of this reply is a practitioner who is not aware of his or her own feelings about the topic, or one who pretends to offer more time and attention than there is to give, and is trying to get away as rapidly as possible.

- Offering Judgmental Responses
  Judgmental responses include several types. For example, those responses that convey approval or disapproval, either verbally or nonverbally, at an inappropriate moment; those that convey advice at a time when it is more important for the patient to make his or her own decision; and responses that are stereotypical: "Adults should know better than to act like children."

- Defensiveness
  When we feel threat to the ego, we respond defensively. Defensiveness indicates a personalization and a refusal to listen carefully to what the patient is saying. A response such as, "You're always late. I've got better

things to do than wait for you, you know" may be true, but does little to solve the patient's tardiness problem.

Values That Underlie Therapeutic Responses

Very often nonhelpful responses are impulsive and reactive, and do not reflect value-based behavior. The values that underlie therapeutic responses were described in Chapter Three. Attitudes such as caring and warmth, respect, compassion and empathy will help interrupt an immature, impulsive response to an emotion-laden communication.

Acceptance of the other person as doing the best he or she can in the moment, and acceptance of the responsibility to be therapeutic in the midst of a chaotic situation are signs of a mature healing professional. These responses emanate from the essential self, not the ego or persona.

Remember that the goal of rehabilitation is to help the patient regain control over his or her life such that independent function at the highest and deepest levels is restored. The role of the practitioner in emotion-laden communication is to ascertain, what is the problem, and whose problem is it?

Identifying Problem Ownership

Learning to send clear messages and to receive accurate messages in intense situations requires identifying who "owns" the problem.[3] Different skills are required for each. For the sake of learning this skill, the rule that applies in every case is: *the person exhibiting the intense emotion is the owner of the problem,* even if he or she is trying desperately to inform you that the problem is really yours.

For example, if the patient is upset with you for being late, and shouts at you as you enter the clinic, "You're late!" you don't have a problem. You just walked into the clinic. The patient who is upset has a problem, even though he might be trying to convince you that you are his problem.

In identifying problem ownership, the person with the emotion "owns" the problem. The first step to resolving the issue is to realize the different skills required depending on who owns the problem. Table 6-1 illustrates the two sets of skills required, active listening and "I" statements.[3]

Emotion-laden exchanges are cluttered with intense feelings, derogatory remarks, apologies, illustrations, etc. In order to sort out the problem, special listening skills are needed to defuse the emotion, and get at the problem. Critical to this method is the resistance of the desire of the unhelpful response to want to "fix" it right away to get rid of the anger or conflict. The alternative is to listen by resisting the quick advice, or the defensive reply.

Active Listening—When the Other Has the Problem

Active listening is a form of therapeutic listening that helps the agitated person with the problem hear clearly what he or she is trying to say. It

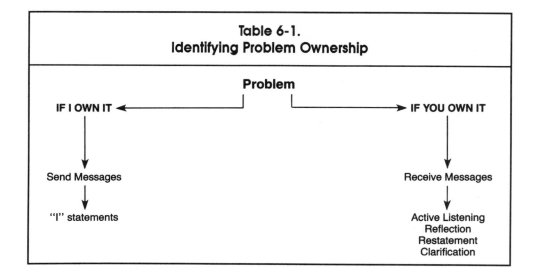

Table 6-1.
Identifying Problem Ownership

involves paraphrasing the speaker's words rather than reacting to them in order to clarify if you have caught the intended meaning. You must suspend your thoughts, and attend exclusively to the words of the other person. *This is not easy,* and requires development as a new skill. In a sense, it requires self transposal, where you work to put yourself in the other person's shoes, to understand rather than judge or defend against. For some it will require great effort to resist responding with a suggestion of what to do, since the desire to fix it for others is so habitual.

Active listening is made up of three different processes:

1. Restatement—repeating the words of the speaker as you have heard them.

    Example: "I get so frustrated that I never have a day free from my back pain."

    Restatement: "You're frustrated because the back pain never leaves you?"

    Restatement can be annoying if not timed appropriately. When done well, it assures the patient that you have, indeed, heard the content of what he or she is saying. The main purpose of restatement is to help the person continue speaking, and should only be used in the *initial phases* of active listening. Once you have reassured the patient that you are hearing his or her words, reflection and clarification become more useful responses.

2. Reflection—Verbalizing both the content and the implied feelings of the sender.

    Example: "This pain has been going on for months. I just can't go on any longer."

    Reflection—"You're exhausted and feeling defeated from the constant pain?"

The purpose of reflection is to express in words the feelings and attitudes sensed behind the words of the sender. This aspect of listening indicates you're hearing more than just the words, you're hearing the emotion behind them. Sometimes we guess incorrectly, but this gives the sender the chance to clarify for us and for him or herself exactly what he or she is feeling. Awareness of feelings is critical to identifying the real problem. When the listener wants to help the sender to examine more extensively both thoughts and feelings, or to focus thoughts and feelings, clarification is used.

3. Clarification—summarizing or simplifying the sender's thoughts and feelings and resolving confused verbalizations into clear, concise statements.

   Example: "When the doctor told me I needed physical therapy, I knew that you would be the person who would help me get rid of my pain. But it's been two weeks now and the pain just keeps coming back. I am afraid that I'll have this pain forever. I'm not sure what it is that I'm supposed to do. Do I just have to live with this or will somebody please help me?"

   Clarification—"When you first came to physical therapy, you thought the pain would be relieved immediately. Now you realize that ridding yourself of the pain is going to take longer than you expected, and is more than a matter of somebody just fixing it?"

   These skills take practice, as does resisting the answer that tends toward "fixing it." The exercises at the end of the chapter will give you an opportunity to practice.

Clear Sending—Use of ``I'' Statements When I Own the Problem

When I feel the emotion and want to communicate to another person that I am upset, clear communication is facilitated when I am congruent. That is, my words clearly match my feelings. I express my feelings with "I" messages rather than the commonly used editorial "they," or "you" or "everyone." First let's look at congruence.

Congruence

Congruence is a term that indicates that the words and the music match. Congruence is present when what I say matches what I do and what I feel. Incongruence appears ingenuine and dishonest, "not ringing true." How often we have been caught in incongruence when someone asks for a compliment: "Well, do you like my new haircut or *not*?" "Well, yes, it's okay I guess." What was felt was less than okay but no one likes to appear rude. When a person is congruent, he or she appears open, honest, genuine, and authentic. Nonverbal cues and tone of voice are consistent with the words spoken.

Congruence requires reflection. Before speaking, you must realize both feelings and thoughts, and reconcile such pulls as wanting not to be hurtful, yet wanting to be honest. A congruent response to the requested compliment might be: "You know, I noticed you had a new haircut, but I believe I liked it better the old way." With this response, the person realizes that you value honesty, and are willing to be honest and can avoid being rude. The message "rings true" and you feel better. More important, the person knows you will resist responses aimed at trying to please others.

Congruence is best conveyed when it is communicated with sensitivity and thought. It should never be used as a rationalization for insensitive and rude "honesty."

"I" Messages

"I" messages are necessary when you feel emotion, you own the problem and you want to get the problem solved. Our tendency is to blame when we feel uncomfortable. An example might be: "You always leave the dirty dishes in the sink! I'm getting sick and tired of cleaning up after you." What is the problem, and whose problem is it?

Well, I'm upset, so the problem is mine, and requires a clearer message than that if I want to get it solved in a helpful way. Using an "I" message, this is the way I would proceed:

"I'm feeling very frustrated. This is the third night in a row that I've found dirty dishes in the sink and I'm tired of doing them for you. Let's talk about this."

With "I" messages, I clearly own my frustration. Then it's up to the other person to respond, hopefully with concern, perhaps even with active listening. Please note, however, that use of an "I" statement does not guarantee that the other person will respond in a helpful way. What it does guarantee is that my feelings will be expressed and I will take responsibility for my upset, rather than blaming someone else. Another person might never get upset over dirty dishes in the sink!

Using "I" statements involves taking a risk. I speak in the first person, I "own" my feelings rather than ignore, disclaim or minimize them. It takes reflective thought to decide what it is that I'm feeling and how it is I can express that. Sending "I" messages tells the other person that you are owning your upset, and both you and he or she are worthy, and capable of solving this problem with appropriate, clear, respectful discussion.

The exercises at the end of the chapter will help you practice this important skill, as well.

Conclusion

Communication that is helpful resists the need to impulsively respond, or to offer quick advice, or a quick solution to a problem. Instead, therapeutic communication strives to clarify the problem, and to assist the person with the problem to solve it for him or herself. When we were children, we needed older adults to fix it for us, to put a bandaid on our bruised knees or our bruised egos. As mature health practitioners, we must unlearn the natural tendency to help by giving advice. We must respect and value the communication process as one more tool in our repertoire of therapeutic responses where we help the other person help him or herself.

Let's return to the case example at the beginning of the chapter. Jonathan and Mrs. Graham are standing in the hallway outside Diane's room, and Mrs. Graham has just let Jonathan have it. What is the problem and whose problem is it?

Clearly it is Mrs. Graham's problem. Jonathan has practiced his therapeutic communication skills, and instead of defending himself responds with, "You're obviously upset and frustrated at the apparent lack of progress on Diane's part, and you believe that is due to my inexperience."

Mrs. Graham says yes and goes on for another few minutes, while Jonathan keeps up with her with active listening responses. Soon she calms down, and, feeling really listened to, she looks at Jonathan and admits that the real problem is that she feels that this is all her fault, and she feels so helpless. Jonathan explores with her what he believes are her choices in dealing with the guilt she feels, and then promises to include her in his therapy sessions to a greater extent tomorrow, so that she can provide minor aspects of treatment in the evenings. Mrs. Graham shakes his hand and thanks him, and agrees to see a counselor to work on her feelings of guilt.

Not all communications will end that amicably, but the majority will end far less amicably if the practitioner responds impulsively or simply reacts. Therapeutic communication is the most useful way to insure a helping response to emotion-laden communication.

References

1. Cassell, EJ: *Talking with Patients.* Volume 1. Cambridge, MA, MIT Press, 1985, p. 4.
2. Kozler, B, Erb, GL: *Fundamentals of Nursing.* Concepts and Procedures. Reading, Mass., Addison-Wesley Publishers, 1979.
3. Munson, PJ, Johnson, RB: *Humanizing Instruction or Helping Your Students Up the Up Staircase.* Chapel Hill, Johnson Self Instructional Package, 1972.

exercises

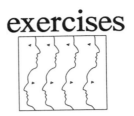

1. Current Patterns

Think of a recent situation in which you felt emotionally upset or frustrated. Describe the situation on paper briefly.

Whose problem was it? If you were upset, it was *your* problem. How did you communicate? Did you communicate at all, or did you swallow it and hope it would go away, or at least change so it was no longer a problem?

What did you communicate, exactly?

How would you change that now, using "I" statements or active listening? Do you think the outcome would have changed if you had used "I" messages or active listening?

Write an "I" statement designed to communicate your upset.

2. Active Listening

Active listening involves restatement (of the words of the sender), reflection (of the words and underlying feelings of the sender) and clarification (summarizes and focuses the sender's message). Practice writing all three types of responses as requested below.

Restatement

Sender

I'm very worried about my shortness of breath.

I used to be able to jog for a whole hour, but now my joints start to ache.

I wish I could swim for 100 laps without getting so tired.

Response from You

You're worried about your shortness of breath?

Reflection

Sender

This pain has been going on for months now. I just wish someone would fix it for me.

Response

Your pain just drags on and you wish someone would help relieve it. Perhaps you're concerned that it will never go away?

Yesterday was a good day, but today I feel the same old way.

It's hard remembering to do my exercises. I want to get better, but it's hard.

Clarification

Sender	*Response*
I wish someone would tell me what's going on with my knees. When I get up in the morning they're fine, but by noon they're swollen and feel tired. I'm too young to be suffering with joint problems. Is this arthritis or what? Do I have to live with this forever?	You're worried that your knee problem might be arthritis, and that you'll never be rid of it?
So when the chiropractor told me I had a curved spine and I had to keep coming back for more adjustments every day I felt that surely there must be something I could do for myself. I got a little frustrated by having so little to do to help myself.	
I almost didn't make it here. I got a horrible headache as I was driving here. The traffic is so stressful in this city. Will it ever end? New cars every day on the road. I don't know if I can keep up driving, with these headaches. Is there anything you can do for me?	

3. "I" Messages

Read each situation and the "you" message (blaming response), then write an "I" message in the third column.

Situation	"You" message	"I" message
The aide has neglected to clean the whirlpool for three days in a row.	What's the matter with you? Are you getting lazy or what?	I'm confused and frustrated. For three days the whirlpool hasn't been cleaned. What's the problem?
Your patient has arrived late and set your schedule back by a half hour all day!	You're late again! Now I'm going to be a half hour behind for the last three treatment sessions.	
The patient seems depressed and has been reluctant to speak up for several days.	You're so quiet lately. Did I do something to make you mad?	

4. Patient/Practitioner Interactions

A series of vignettes follows. Divide up into groups of three, where one person is the health professional, one person is the patient and one person is the observer.

Role play the first vignette for five minutes or so, or until an appropriate place to stop occurs. The observer should have in hand a copy of the "Patient/Practitioner Interaction Check List" which follows Vignette 4. At the conclusion of the vignette, the observer asks the patient how he or she is feeling, then asks the practitioner the same question. The observer then gives the practitioner feedback as recorded on the check list. At the end of the first round (approximately 15 minutes), remain in the same group of three, but exchange roles and repeat the same vignette, utilizing the same process. Repeat for the third time before moving on to a new vignette. After all three of you have role played the practitioner, discuss the experience among yourselves. Take a risk and give each other helpful feedback, negative and positive, about your communication skills. Journal about the experience focusing on what it felt like to be the therapist, to be the patient, to be the observer giving negative feedback to a classmate or colleague.

Vignettes

Each person playing a role should see the description for that role *only*. Read the brief description and then act out the part as you would if it were happening to you. These vignettes are written for the role of physical therapist, but feel free to alter the descriptions to make them more applicable to the role which you are preparing for in your education if it is not physical therapy.

Vignette 1

Physical Therapist

You've been working with this patient who is wheelchair bound for four months. The last three weeks the two of you have focused on the patient's discharge home. The patient seems both pleased to be returning home, but also anxious. You notice lately that the patient is short-tempered and cuts people off who try to help. You hate conflict and want to avoid it at all costs.

Patient

You are wheelchair bound and have been working in physical therapy for four months with the same therapist. The last three weeks the two of you have focused on your discharge home. You've begun to be very anxious about separating from the rehabilitation center and are experiencing intermittent episodes of chest pain. You're afraid to tell anyone about this, for you fear they will discount your symptoms and label you as over dependent, and actually you're afraid that they might be right. You're exhausted, as you haven't slept more than one or two hours for the past three nights. You decide to confide your fears to your physical therapist, but you're feeling very exhausted and defensive. You decide to just blurt it all out and hope that your therapist will understand.

Vignette 2
Physical Therapist

You are the therapist for a cerebral palsied children's program. One mother brings her child three times a week to your center and stays and watches you treat her daughter along with the other children. This child is African American, and several races are represented at the center. You are Caucasian. This center is the only place where children with cerebral palsy can get treatment in this small town.

Patient's Mother

You are the mother of a child with cerebral palsy. You bring your child to physical therapy at the rehabilitation center in your small town three times each week and wait while she receives treatment. You notice that the physical therapist seems to spend less time with your daughter than she spends with two other children. You are African American and the others are Caucasian, as is the physical therapist. You've decided to confront the therapist with your suspicions. You're angry and hurt, but you fear that if you say the wrong thing, your daughter will be treated even less than before. This is the only center in town that offers treatment for your child. This is not the first time you've felt that you and your family were being discriminated against because of your race.

Vignette 3
Physical Therapist

Your 20-year-old patient who had minor knee surgery a week ago is still complaining of pain. He keeps his knee elevated with ice, hates to do exercises, screams with pain and uses his crutches only with assistance to go to the bathroom. The surgeon is anxious to discharge the patient home, but you're convinced that he is not ready, and will surely fall. He has ten stairs to climb just to get from the sidewalk to the front door of his house. You're subconsciously afraid that your lack of experience in caring for patients with knee surgery has contribute to his poor recovery, so you're feeling guilty.

Patient

You have just had knee surgery one week ago and are experiencing a lot of postoperative pain. You're protecting your knee, keeping it very still so it will heal faster and hurt less. Your physical therapist seems to think you should have been discharged home days ago and is frustrated with your oversensitivity to the pain. You've never had surgery before, and no one really prepared you for this experience. You're afraid you'll be discharged tomorrow, and you feel very shaky with your crutches. You have no idea how you'll climb up the ten steps to your front porch, let alone the 15 to your bedroom. You're upset with yourself for being afraid, you hurt, you're fearful of being thrown out in the cold with no help. You decide to talk to your therapist before physical therapy today. You feel angry at her for putting you in this position.

Vignette 4
Physical Therapist

You are with a private practice assigned to cover the patient care needs at a nursing home and, although you love the patients and enjoy the interaction with them, you realize that much of their functional activity has to be supervised by the nursing staff when you are not there. The nurses love the patients also, but they are short-staffed. They are constantly asking you to help them with nursing functions while you are doing therapy, and you cooperate but are becoming more and more frustrated. You decide to talk to the head nurse about this after you discuss one of your patients who needs to be ambulated three times a shift to build endurance. You approach the nurse as she is making out her daily census report.

Nurse

You are in charge of a unit of elderly patients and you are understaffed. The administrator has been criticizing you for inefficiency, and you feel she is being unrealistic in her demands on you. Secretly you fear that if one more thing goes wrong you are likely to lose your job. The physical therapist has asked to see you, and you are angry at her because she seems to make more work for your nurses so that their nursing tasks do not get completed. The physical therapist is always asking the nurses to dangle patients or help ambulate them; you think they should hire another therapist and let your nurses do nursing care.

Journaling

At the conclusion of the exercises, journal your feelings about this new form of communicating. How do you feel about its usefulness? Do you believe you will be able to develop skill in using "I" statements? Are you willing to practice at home? How about active listening skills? Make a commitment to practice using these skills at least once each day until you believe you've developed some skill, and remember that this form of communication is now a choice for you in any situation.

Patient/Practitioner Interaction Check List

The observer in the triad responds to these questions during each role play situation, and the uses this information to give feedback to the practitioner about his or her therapeutic communication.

How well did the practitioner:

1. Attend to the patient's (or nurse's) emotional state and feelings?

2. Identify what the problem was and who had the problem?

3. Use reflection and clarifying responses during active listening, use "I" statements when he or she owned the problem?

4. Use open-ended questions and statements to encourage the patient to talk more?

5. Remain silent when appropriate?

6. Respond to the patient with signs of sympathy and self transposal?

7. Avoid judging, defensive or blaming statements?

8. How could the therapist improve communication next time?

chapter seven

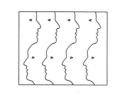

ASSERTIVENESS SKILLS

Objectives

1. To identify the importance of using assertive communication in healing interactions.
2. To distinguish between nonassertive, assertive and aggressive communication.
3. To point out that there are situations in which each person tends to give up personal power.
4. To identify the rights we all share as human beings.
5. To offer the opportunity to contract for changing negative, reactive behavior to positive, assertive behavior.

Assertiveness Training

In the previous chapter we learned a new way of communicating in intense or emotional moments. This chapter expands on the skills previously learned, and teaches a way of communicating that will improve one's sense of personal power and self-esteem in situations where stress would have us give up that power.

Let's begin with a case example:

Sheila Lester, registered nurse, was standing at the nurses' station reading her patient's chart before going into the patient's room to give her treatment. The patient's physician came to the station and was searching for the chart. When he saw that Sheila was reading it, he turned to her and said, "Give me the chart, Honey; that's my patient and I have to see her now." Sheila felt as if she were being treated in a nonprofessional way, to say the least. She felt her heart begin to race, she knew she was blushing, and she realized that she felt degraded and humiliated. Before she could stop herself, she turned to the physician and shouted, "My name is not Honey, and this is my patient, as well!" The physician looked up with amusement and returned, "Well, well; what is your name then, Honey?" Sheila felt as if the battle were lost, and put the chart down and walked away in anger.

Assertiveness training has become well-known in the past decade and many people claim its benefits as a communication skill, but it also carries a negative connotation in some circles. Images of the "uppity" woman or the aggressive man come to view. These images result from our socialization, from the messages we heard from our parents as we grew up. As rambunctious children, many of us were taught that we should "know our place" and practice humility. As we grew older, we heard other messages, rules such as "Children should be seen and not heard"; "Go to your room until you can come out with a smile on your face!"; "If you can't say something nice, don't say anything at all"; and "Women belong in the supportive role to their husbands." The accumulative effect, especially on women who suffer from low self-esteem, can result in communication that is not healthy or healing in nature. Following all those rules results in multiple unhealthy behaviors: the bottling up of genuine emotion, the repression of feelings over time that often results in stress-related illness, passive-aggressive silence or manipulation, and inappropriate outbursts of anger, defensiveness and frustration.

The Challenge of Communicating Wisely in Health Care

Health care calls for a great deal of practice when dealing with fellow practitioners who are often working under stress and when dealing with patients and their families who are feeling intensely vulnerable. Emotional communication, including anger, is very prevalent in the practice of health care. There are many situations that occur daily in which a person is stimulated to react either in anger or in giving up personal power and feeling helpless.

Gender Differences

Women predominate in all of the health professions except medicine and surgery. However, we live in an evolving society that has been, and continues to be, essentially male-dominated and patriarchal. In spite of the fact that health care consists of much more than physician care, medicine was created by men to be practiced by men. Nurses, who are predominantly women, feel especially affected by this disparate power structure. In a study conducted by Friedman on nurse-physician relationships, nurses reported that they had to deal with: 1) condescending attitudes, 2) lack of respect as either a person or a professional, 3) public humiliation as physicians rant and rave in front of patients, families or anyone who will listen, 4) temper tantrums, 5) scapegoating (nurses are blamed for everything that goes wrong), 6) failure to read nurses' notes or listen to nurses' suggestions, 7) refusal to share information about the patient, and 8) frequent public disparaging remarks.[1]

The continuum of insensitive behavior issuing from people in power to those in less powerful positions can run from poor taste and bad manners to outright sexist abuse and harassment. The sources of verbal abuse to nurses described in the Friedman article were primarily physicians, then patients' families and lastly, the nurse's supervisor.[1] So although it is true to point out that part of the power struggle in health care has to do with the difficulties in our culture of men and women relating equally with each other, it is not as simple as that.

As much as all children are alike, developmentalists have shown us that boys and girls are different in the way they are treated by adults, in their goals and ideals, in the way they see their place in the world, in the way they make decisions about right and wrong. But all people have a genderless essential self, a core identity that is good that underlies the public self or persona and the ego. All people have the natural desire to become more, to grow, to learn, to increase self-esteem, to have influence and to feel capable and able to facilitate change for the better. People in health care, both men and women, for the most part, want to help others, to change conditions of illness and pain, or inability to function fully as a human being in the world. To help in healing ways, one must exercise personal and professional power for the good. The goal must be to mature beyond the need for the ego to defend itself, and to reach down to the essential self, where we are confident of our personal rights and assured of our equality, and from where we can communicate with empathy and understanding.

Exercising Our Personal Power

In Section One we learned that how we feel about ourselves has everything to do with how we view the world and how we view other people. How we feel about our own self-worth also is directly connected to how much personal power we feel we have, and how we use that power.

Webster defines *power* as a possession of control, authority or influence over another; the ability to act or produce an effect; legal or official authority, capacity or right; physical might; or political control or influence.[2] Notice that power is a neutral term, having neither positive nor negative value connotations. If we want to facilitate change, make the world better, we have to learn how to exercise power.

Women in our society have been taught to play a role secondary to or supportive of men. Men have been taught to seek out and expect the support of women. But we are all born equal. We learn to give up our power. Some beliefs that we develop that result in a giving up of personal power include the following.

1. I'm not as important as the other person (often the physician).
2. I am lucky to be treated with respect by others (those in authority).
3. I have years of training and experience, but they still do not compare to medical school.
4. I must act in ways that indicate I know my place so that I can keep my job, keep referrals coming, keep peace for others' sake.
5. When criticized by a superior, I must not respond, but agree in order to save face and avoid further criticism.
6. My needs are not as important as others'.

Some situations seem inherently more apt to stimulate stress than others, thus we can predict that we might be tempted to give up power when we find ourselves required to respond in the midst of one. Ten such situations that cause stress for some or all of us include:

1. Command—someone orders us to do something.
2. Anger—includes name-calling, using obscenities, shouting.
3. Criticism—someone judges us as being less than adequate.
4. Unresponsiveness—indifference to us, or to our request.
5. Depression—a feeling of gloom in another, extreme sadness.
6. Impulsivity—someone flies off the handle, acts crazy.
7. Affection—someone expresses love and affection, or asks us for it.
8. Making mistakes—fear that you cannot make a mistake; feeling as if you must always have the right answer.
9. Sexual content—someone makes an overt or covert sexual comment or sexual advance.
10. Pain—feelings of wanting to flee in the face of pain.

Personal Rights

Thoughts or beliefs developed even before we could talk lead to feelings (rational or not) which then lead to behavior, or reactions. Everyone is entitled to act assertively and to express honest thoughts, feelings and beliefs. Assertiveness training teaches us that we have a choice of communicating in a way that allows us to convey our thoughts and feelings with tact and respect for others and honor for ourselves. As human beings, each one of us has the right to:

• be treated with respect

- have needs and to have those needs be as important as other people's needs. We have the right to ask (not demand) that other people respond to our needs and to decide if we want to respond to others' needs
- have feelings and express those feelings in ways that do not violate the dignity of others
- change our minds
- determine our own priorities
- ask for what we want
- refuse without making excuses
- form our own opinions and express them, and to have no opinion at all on a certain topic
- give and receive information as fellow health professionals
- act in the best interests of the patient.[3]

When we allow our rights to be overlooked, we assume a dependent role which lowers self-esteem and fosters nonassertive behavior. Recognizing that we have rights is the first step in the cognitive retraining that is essential to assertiveness.

Assertiveness

What, exactly, is assertiveness? The concept of assertive behavior can best be described in comparison to what it is not: nonassertive (passive) and aggressive behavior.

Non-Assertive Behavior

Failing to get your point across by remaining quiet or passive. Perceived by others to be weak, easily taken advantage of, manipulated.

Key message conveyed: I don't count; my feelings are not as important as yours.

Aggressive Behavior

Getting your point across but perceived by others as hostile, angry, offensive, sarcastic or humiliating.

Key message conveyed: This is what is true. Any reasonable person would agree. You are stupid to disagree. What I want is most important, what you want, feel or think does not matter.

Assertive Behavior

Getting your point across without offending others. Direct, congruent expression of thoughts, feelings, beliefs and opinions in a nonoffensive way.

Key message conveyed: This is how I view the situation. This is what I think and feel at this moment.

Alberti and Emmons[4] list ten key elements to assertive behavior:

1. Self expressive
2. Respectful of the rights of others
3. Honest

4. Direct and firm
5. Equalizing; benefiting both self and relationship
6. Verbally appropriate, including the content of the message (feelings, rights, facts, opinions, requests, limits)
7. Nonverbally appropriate, including the style of the message (eye contact, voice posture, facial expression, gestures, distance, timing, fluency, listening)
8. Appropriate for the person and the situation; not universal
9. Socially responsible
10. Learned, not inborn (p. 34)

Examples of Assertive Responses

Many of us have found ourselves in the situation when, dining out, we order our meal and something happens to make it less acceptable than we had expected. We find ourselves in a situation where we feel it is necessary to speak up in order to enjoy the meal that we've requested. Let's say that the dinner is completely cold. What are our choices in this situation?

- Passive—Say nothing at all. When the waitress asks, "How's your dinner?" we respond, "Fine." (The person we're dining with, however, receives the brunt of our hostility all evening).

- Aggressive—Stand up, shout for the waitress or waiter, and say in a loud and angry voice, "This meal is ice cold. I'm willing to pay good money for a good dinner, but you have the nerve to bring me a meal that has been sitting around for half an hour, and I resent it. Take this meal back immediately and bring me some hot food."

- Assertive—Motion for the waiter, state calmly that your food has become cold and request that it be heated and brought back to you as quickly as possible.

Upon comparison, it's easy to value assertive communication as superior to the other two modes. Difficulty acting assertively in appropriate situations with any consistency stems from the real or perceived threat of rejection, anger or disapproval. Often this reluctance to be assertive is based more on habit and subconscious fears that we learned long ago, and that now guide our responses in an automatic way. Assertiveness helps us realize that we have a real choice to stand up for ourselves and to hold onto our power in difficult situations. Why in the world would anyone sit and eat a cold dinner while not enjoying it, and be willing to pay for it? What is the fear behind speaking up to ask for your rights? For many of us it is simply a matter of overlearning the dictate, "Don't make waves, don't cause a fuss, don't do anything that will bring attention to yourself." Behind this admonition is the basic feeling that other's rights are more important than mine; that I don't count.

Types of Assertive Responses

There are eight types of assertive responses that can benefit us in the practice of health care and in our day-to-day interactions:

1. Being confrontive
2. Saying no
3. Making requests
4. Expressing opinions
5. Initiating conversation
6. Disclosing self
7. Expressing affection
8. Entering a room of strangers, willing to get to know others and allowing ourselves to be known

The first two areas can be described as assertive responses that express what commonly appear to be negative emotions; the next three are emotionally neutral responses that are task specific, and the last four call for expressing positive emotions. In the exercises, you will be given the opportunity to draft assertive, passive and aggressive responses to each situation.

Attribution and the Desire to Act Assertively

A person can be quite knowledgeable about assertiveness but will not think to use these skills for any number of reasons. For example, if one believes that no matter what is done, the attempt will end in failure, assertiveness does not seem important. This problematic way of thinking illustrates one aspect of attribution theory.[5]

The following exercise will help you discover the nature of your attributions, or how your lenses are set today.[6]

Put yourself in a time when you've done a project that was highly praised. What did you do? Who praised you? How did you feel? How did this influence future activities? Write down one major *cause* of your success.

1. Is the cause due to something about you, or due to something outside of you?
   Internal 1   2   3   4   5   6   7 External
   Inside you   Other resources

2. Is the cause something that will remain stable or be only temporary?
   Lasting 1   2   3   4   5   6   7 Temporary
   (Stable)   (Unstable)
   Constant (IQ)   Changing (weather)

3. Do you see this cause as something you can control or is this beyond your control?
   Controllable 1   2   3   4   5   6   7 Uncontrollable
   (Whether I study or not)   (Other person's mood)

    Now, think of a time when you have experienced a failure, for example, given an important talk and the audience reacts negatively, or cooked a meal that no one liked. Write down one major *cause*.

4. Is the cause due to something about you or something outside of you?
   Internal 1   2   3   4   5   6   7 External

5. Is the cause something that will remain stable or be only temporary or changing?
   Lasting 1   2   3   4   5   6   7 Temporary
   (Stable)   (Unstable)

6. Do you see this cause as something you can control or is this beyond your control?
   Controllable 1   2   3   4   5   6   7 Uncontrollable

Now chart your numbers on the following grid:

	Success	Failure
Internal/External		
Stable/Unstable		
Control/Uncontrol		

    How likely are you to experience the same outcome in the future?

Success:
Highly likely 1   2   3   4   5   6   7 Unlikely

Failure:
Highly likely 1   2   3   4   5   6   7 Unlikely

    Attribution theory describes one way that a person's lenses are set. An attribution is the cause we give to an outcome we experience. How we view outcomes, as successful or failing, is critical in determining future actions. The three causes of success or failure are the *locus* (due to something inside or outside of me), *stability* (changing or constant) and *controllability* (not a fixed trait, but something I can affect).

Attributions that we assign to outcomes have a great deal to do with how we think about ourselves, or relate directly to how our lenses are set with regard to self esteem. If we have *good self esteem,* we are likely to attribute the cause of our successes to something *inside of ourselves,* something that is *stable* or *controllable.* If we have low self esteem, we see our successes as due to forces outside of ourselves that are unstable and uncontrollable like luck or the difficulty of the task. In other words, with high self esteem, we choose to believe we are going to succeed directly because of our actions, and if we fail, it is not because of a fixed internal trait (we have low ability or a poor personality), but because of circumstances that can change if we apply a different, more successful strategy to the task. In summary, when failure is attributed to stable, external and uncontrollable events, there is little we can do to affect change and we are unlikely to use assertiveness or any other strategy to get the job done. This is a loser's or victim's "script."

It is important to describe the nature of success and failure in ways that allow success to be judged realistically and over the long term.[7] The most adaptive attributions, according to Curtis,[8] occur when success is defined in other than all-or-nothing terms, are realistic in the circumstances and are attributed to one's personal ability, effort or good judgment. In health care many frustrating situations are unlikely to change, but we can change how we think about them and how we deal with them to experience success over the long term. If success is seen as having all patients be discharged from our care fully cured, or have Medicare pay for 100% of treatment in 100% of eligible cases, few practitioners would ever feel as if they succeeded. Compromise, realistic expectations and acceptance of long term strategies are necessary, along with avoiding dualistic right/wrong judgments.

In sum, we must change the way we define failure and think about the causes of failure in order for assertiveness to be useful and successful. If we believe failure is attributed to external events that are uncontrollable and stable, we will be unlikely to use assertiveness. But if we reframe our thoughts, decide that our goal might have been a little too unrealistic, and decide to employ another strategy to work for success, assertiveness can be a useful tool to solve problems.

Learning to Act Assertively

Assertive behavior is not inborn; it is a skill, and to develop it requires learning five new behaviors:[4]

1. Recognize situations in which you are tempted to become passive or aggressive in your communication. Develop the skill of observing yourself. Be conscious of situations where you automatically give up your power,

have irrational thoughts that do not relate to the present moment, feel the necessity to put the other person down.

2. Recognize when you are tempted to attribute fear of failure to forces that are uncontrollable and stable. Challenge yourself to think of a strategy to replace feelings of hopelessness or negativity.

3. Replace these old thought patterns with different thoughts. Cognitively interrupt the old thought patterns of, "You're right, I'm no good." or, "How dare you attack me, you arrogant fool?" or "It's no use!" Alone, or with another trusted person,
   a) discuss the nature of the situation that aroused the emotion
   b) confront the tendency to react passively or aggressively
   c) identify the belief that lies behind your reaction
   d) challenge the erroneous belief with a counteracting right.

4. Practice thinking new thoughts as a first step in changing the feelings that go with the old thoughts, thus deflating the energy behind the old reaction.

5. Practice the new behavior that goes along with the ownership of the right. Be assertive.

How might Sheila, the nurse in the example at the beginning of the chapter, communicate assertively? Well, Chapter Six taught one aspect of assertive communication, the use of "I" statements. This mode of communicating transforms an aggressive, blaming or accusatory response to an assertive, responsible and clear expression of feeling, essentially telling the other person the effect that his or her behavior has on you. In many cases, an "I" statement alone initially is sufficient to get your assertive message across. The situation Sheila found herself in calls for a confrontive assertion. Sheila feels diminished, less than a colleague, more like a slave being asked to do the master's bidding. Her feeling response is anger at being treated so poorly, and her initial reaction is to be angry. When her anger does not get her what she wants, the messages in her head revert to, "See. You're just not as good as the physician. Your rights are not important here." She gives up and walks away in frustration. What she hoped for was a collegial relationship with the physician, as both of them carry out their clinical responsibilities with the patient. This calls for a confrontive response aimed at helping her avoid becoming aggressive in anger, and avoid passively giving up her power to silently comply with the physician's rude request.

First Sheila must be aware of her feelings in the situation, her tendency to react in anger and give up her power. She must be aware of how she attributes possible outcomes to any behavior in this situation. Next she must be aware of the messages she gives herself and challenge the negative thoughts with more affirming, positive thoughts that confirm her rights as a human being. Then she is ready to respond with an assertive reply aimed at exercising her right to express her honest thoughts, feelings and beliefs around this situation. One format for an effective response is the DESC response.

DESC Response as a Format for Assertive Communication

The DESC format described by Bower and Bower[8] incorporates "I" statements but expands them and is useful when a more detailed interaction is required to get the other person's attention to your point of view.
DESC is an acronym for:

D—Describe the situation
E—Express your feelings about the situation: "I feel _____."
S—Specify the change you want: "I'd like for you to _____."
C—Consequences. Identify the results that will occur: "In that way _____."

Let's compose a DESC response for Sheila in the situation outlined at the beginning of the chapter:

D—Yes, Dr. Dutton, I realize that this is your patient. She's my patient as well; I'm her nurse.
E—My name is Sheila Lester. When you call me "Honey" it demeans me and I don't appreciate it.
S—I'd like you to call me Sheila or Ms. Lester because I'd like to discuss this patient with you as a colleague would. And I would like you to treat me as a colleague.
C—In that way I feel the patient will receive better care because we are working together with her in a more respectful and collegial way.

Sheila took a big risk with this physician by speaking up to tell him how his behavior made her feel. She must have trusted that this was a risk worth taking. We would hope that the physician would respond in a mature way, and treat her request with respect. Assertive communication does not guarantee this, however, as we'll discuss in a moment.

Sometimes you know that the risk is not well-placed. An alternative to the DESC confrontation is the DISC confrontation, which is used when you are confronting a person who will not care what you feel, so you eliminate the expression of feeling and substitute I for Indicate, indicating the problem the behavior is causing. DESC and DISC are really just amplifications of the effective "I" statement. But using them in a practiced, disciplined way provides an opportunity to erase an old, ineffective way of responding by replacing it with an assertive response.

An illustration of the DISC response for a physical therapist would be:

A powerful physician refers a patient with low back pain to you, a physical therapist, and specifically orders:

Evaluate and treat with heat and massage. No exercise, no mobilization.

Upon evaluation you realize that this back pain is the result of an acute muscle spasm which occurred recently and was facilitated by poor body mechanics and weak extensor muscles. Your professional knowledge requires that you treat with ice and teach exercises to relax the current problem and prevent recurrence.

Your DISC confrontation might go something like this:

D—I'd like to talk with you about Mr. Doughty's back problem.

I—Your physical therapy referral for heat and massage is a logical place to start for a chronic problem, but my examination reveals this to be an acute spasm which the literature indicates responds faster and more effectively to ice. Likewise, his back extensor and abdominal muscles are quite weak, and he needs gentle relaxation exercise to reduce the spasm and eventual instruction in proper body mechanics.

S—I'd like for you to approve my plan to treat with ice and massage, then follow with gentle pelvic tilt and bridging exercises to tolerance to release the spasm, and eventually teach him stretching and strengthening exercises and proper body mechanics to prevent recurrence.

C—That way perhaps we can help him recover, and get him strong enough and wise enough to keep him from reinjuring himself.

Organizing your thoughts will be more difficult, at first, and so the exercises for this chapter will provide practice following this four step method by writing out your response to a past situation that was particularly difficult for you.

You're probably wondering how you'll learn to respond quickly and on the spot with such a detailed DISC or DESC format when an assertive response is indicated. At first you will not be so organized. The most you can hope for is to recognize your feelings, avoid giving up your power angrily or passively, and buy time before responding at all. Eventually, however, it will become second nature to speak up with an "I" statement or a DESC response.

Assertively Dealing With Anger

Every once in awhile you will have to deal with an angry, defensive person. Feeling trapped in another's lashing out usually stimulates a flight or fight response, or passive or aggressive behavior. The ego is stimulated into defending itself, or the ego caves in to fear and wants to run away. In the previous chapter we learned to use active listening when the other person has the emotional outburst; this continues to be the most effective response in an assertive mode. Using active listening skills to help the person defuse the energy behind the outburst, which is most often secondary to fear, allows you then to use "I" statements to offer your assertive response. In other words, be a Teflon sponge; absorb the emotion by using restatement, reflection and clarification, and let it slide off of you.

What people are most asking for is recognition and understanding. Active listening gives you the chance to stand still and offer a therapeutic response which will increase the chances for a positive outcome to the interchange. Once emotions have been dissipated, offer your assertive point of view and offer to work together to solve the problem.[9]

Benefits of Assertiveness

There are several benefits to using assertive behavior:
- it is our ethical and healing responsibility
- it increases our self respect
- it increases our self control
- it improves self confidence
- it helps us develop more emotionally satisfying relationships with others
- it increases the likelihood that everyone's needs will be met
- it allows us to exercise our personal rights without denying the rights of others.

> To exercise our personal rights relates to competency as a citizen, as a consumer, as a member of an organization or school or work group, as a participant in public events to express opinions, to work for change, to respond to violations of one's own rights or those of others.[4,p.26]

In the health professions, we must work side by side with colleagues, helping our patients regain their feelings of confidence and ability to function independently in the world. In order to make sure this happens, everyone's rights become important, and the exercise of those rights is critical to the healing process.

Common Myths About Assertiveness

As valuable as assertive communication is, there are some common myths that accompany this process:

1. If I speak up with assertiveness, others will like what I say, and do what I ask.

   Using assertive communication is no guarantee for anything, except that you have expressed yourself with dignity, honesty and with regard for others. How others respond to you is always a question, and has much to do with the other person. Most important, you never have the right to violate another person's rights, even when you use assertiveness.

2. All I have to do is say the assertive words and I will be perceived as being assertive.

   Assertive words are critical to an assertive message. But assertive words spoken passively or aggressively destroy the basic message of assertiveness. The posture of assertiveness is an appropriate tone of voice, a steady voice, open posture and good eye contact.

3. Once I learn assertiveness skills, I must use them all the time in every situation that tends to make me feel powerless.

There are times when the best assertive response is to simply walk away and say nothing. One good example is deciding not to retaliate to an aggressive person. Then it is best to say nothing. Always remember, you are free to choose not to assert yourself in a situation. Ask yourself:

How important is this situation to me?

How am I likely to feel afterwards if I don't assert myself?

What will the cost be to assert myself now? Is it worth it?

4. One assertive reply is all that's needed.

The first assertive response is the easiest. It's the "comeback" response that even's more difficult. People will argue with your assertive response and try to get you to give up your power in spite of your effectiveness. For example, saying no when you mean no often takes several repeats of the no, and you may decide to end the conversation with, "Don't try to make me feel guilty. I told you I care about you, but I will not say yes this time. I said no; I mean no. End of discussion."

The exercises begin with self awareness about your own tendencies to respond passively or aggressively in certain situations. They proceed into opportunities for you to practice assertive communication with your classmates in role playing situations. Don't forget to journal about the impact that the readings and exercises have on you. How does all of this make you feel? The exercises conclude with the opportunity for you to negotiate a personal contract for change, for to truly change behavior that has been practiced for many years takes more than good intentions, it takes a promise. And for some of you, at first your new behavior will feel awkward and ingenuine. My advice is, fake it until you make it. Rarely will I suggest ingenuineness, but for many of us, we've overlearned the feelings that accompany low self-esteem, and need to dramatically break up harmful, reactive behaviors to false beliefs. Ideally we could all experience the necessary inner transformations quickly and congruently. Life is a bit more complex than that. So, start the process from outside-in rather than from inside-out. The goal is the same. The outer behavior, as inauthentic as it feels, for example, to be equal to a physician, is still in everyone's best interest. Act as if you have every one of those rights listed above, and eventually you will accept it as the truth. And it is!

References

1. Friedman, FB: A nurse's guide to the care and handling of MDs. *RN,* March, 1982, pp. 39-43.
2. *Webster's Seventh New Collegiate Dictionary.* Springfield, MA, G. & C. Merriam Co., 1963.
3. Chenevert, M: *STAT—Special Techniques in Assertiveness Training for Women in Health Professions.* St. Louis, C.V. Mosby, 1978.
4. Alberti, RE, Emmons, ML: *Your Perfect Right.* (5th ed.) San Luis Obispo, Impact Publishers, 1986.
5. Anderson, C, Jennings, DL: When experiences of failure promote expectations of success: The impact of attributing failure to ineffective strategies. *Journal of Personality,* 48:393-407, 1980.
6. Curtis, K. Personal communication.
7. Weiner, B: Attribution theory and attributional therapy: Some theoretical observations and suggestions. *British Journal of Clinical Psychology,* 27:93-104, 1988.
8. Curtis, K: Altering beliefs about the importance of strategy: and attributional intervention. *Journal of Applied Social Psychology,* 22:953-972, 1992.
9. Bower, SA, Bower, GH: *Asserting Yourself.* Reading, MA, Addison Wesley, 1976.
10. Silber, M: Managing confrontations: once more into the breach. *Nursing Management,* 15:54-58, April, 1984.
11. Gawain, S: *Living in the Light.* San Rafael, CA, New World Library, 1986.

exercises

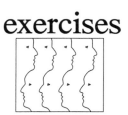

1. My Rights as a Person

When we hear terrifying stories of people's inhumanity to each other, we're often moved to righteous indignation. For example, none of us can hear recountings from holocaust victims without cringing with horror. Likewise, prisoner of war stories move us to anger and outrage. Human beings deserve to be treated in certain ways simply because we are human. What rights do we have, as human beings? What does each human being deserve, simply by virtue of the fact that he or she is a person, alive on this earth? Make a list of the basic rights of all human beings.

Now reflect on that list in your journal. Do you act in ways that are consistent with your beliefs about your rights? Are there certain rights that you fail to claim for yourself? If so, why is that?

How does this list change when a human being becomes ill or disabled? Journal about the rights of people who are ill or in need of health care.

2. Self-Awareness—Assertiveness Inventory

Complete the Assertiveness Inventory from Alberti and Emmons' *Your Perfect Right*.[4] As directed at the bottom of the survey, circle the three statements that most often result in your giving up your power and becoming passive, or so angry that you become aggressive.

1. Look at your responses to questions 1, 2, 4, 5, 6, 7, 9, 10, 11, 12, 14, 15, 16, 17, 18, 19, 21, 22, 24, 25, 27, 28, 30, and 35. These questions are oriented toward nonassertive behavior. Are you rarely speaking up for yourself? Or is there one situation that gives you more problem than the others? If so, journal about it starting with the earliest memories you have about that incident.

2. Look at your responses to questions 3, 8, 13, 20, 23, 26, 29, 31, 32, 33, and 34. These questions are oriented toward aggressive behavior. Are you pushing others around more than you realized? Does one question give you more trouble than the others? Again, journal about it, as above.

3. Few people are assertive all the time, aggressive all the time or passive all the time. The situation often dictates the response. On rereading your total responses, do you see a pattern? Do you favor one way of responding over the others? Draw some conclusions about yourself from the inventory and journal about them. Which situations cause you most trouble? Which situations do you handle with no trouble at all? Why is that?

4. Can you identify obstacles that stand in the way of asserting yourself confidentially? What beliefs do you hold about yourself and the world that make it difficult, or easy to assert yourself? What is the worst thing that could happen? Journal about your learning.

5. Ask family members and trusted friends to give you honest and specific feedback about their observations of your behavior under stress. Do you show patterns of passivity or aggressiveness? Ask them to illustrate their points with examples. Resist the natural desire to defend yourself as they respond. Just listen, and take notes, then journal about what you learned, and about your feelings.

Alberti and Emmons: *Your Perfect Right* 2nd ed. Impact Publishers, San Luis Obispo, CA, 1974.

Assertiveness Inventory

The following questions will be helpful in assessing your assertiveness. Be honest in your responses. All you have to do is draw a circle around the number that describes you best. For some questions the assertive end of the scale is at 0, for others at 4. Key: 0 means *no* or *never*; 1 means *somewhat* or *sometimes*; 2 means *average*; 3 means *usually* or *a good deal*; and 4 means *practically always* or *entirely*.

1. When a person is highly unfair, do you call it to his or her attention?. 0 1 2 3 4
2. Do you find it difficult to make decisions?. 0 1 2 3 4
3. Are you openly critical of others' ideas, opinions, behavior?. 0 1 2 3 4
4. Do you speak out in protest when someone takes your place in line?. 0 1 2 3 4
5. Do you often avoid people or situations for fear of embarrassment?. 0 1 2 3 4
6. Do you usually have confidence in your own judgment?. 0 1 2 3 4
7. Do you insist that your spouse or roommate take on a fair share of household 0 1 2 3 4
   chores?. . . . .
8. Are you prone to "fly off the handle"?. 0 1 2 3 4
9. When a salesperson makes an effort, do you find it hard to say "No" even 0 1 2 3 4
   though the merchandise is not really what you want?. . . . .
10. When a latecomer is waited on before you are, do you call attention to the 0 1 2 3 4
    situation?. . . . .
11. Are you reluctant to speak up in a discussion or debate?. 0 1 2 3 4
12. If a person has borrowed money for a book, garment, (thing of value) and is 0 1 2 3 4
    overdue in returning it, do you mention it?. . . . .
13. Do you continue to pursue an argument after the other person has had enough? 0 1 2 3 4
14. Do you generally express what you feel?. 0 1 2 3 4
15. Are you disturbed if someone watches you at work?. 0 1 2 3 4
16. If someone seems kicking or bumping your chair in a movie or a lecture, do you 0 1 2 3 4
    ask the person to stop?. . . . .
17. Do you find it difficult to keep eye contact when talking to another person?. . 0 1 2 3 4
18. In a good restaurant, when your meal is improperly prepared or served, do you 0 1 2 3 4
    ask the waiter/waitress to correct the situation?. . . . .
19. When you discover merchandise is faulty, do you return it for an adjustment?. 0 1 2 3 4
20. Do you show your anger by name-calling or obscenities?. 0 1 2 3 4
21. Do you try to be a wallflower or a piece of the furniture in social situations?. 0 1 2 3 4
22. Do you insist that your landlord (mechanic, repairperson, etc.) make repairs, 0 1 2 3 4
    adjustment or replacements which are his or her responsibility?. . . . .
23. Do you often step in and make decisions for others?. 0 1 2 3 4
24. Are you able to openly express love and affection?. 0 1 2 3 4
25. Are you able to ask your friends for small favors or help?. 0 1 2 3 4
26. Do you think you always have the right answer?. 0 1 2 3 4
27. When you differ with a person you respect, are you able to speak up for your 0 1 2 3 4
    own viewpoint?. . . . .
28. Are you able to refuse unreasonable requests made by friends?. 0 1 2 3 4
29. Do you have difficulty complimenting or praising others?. 0 1 2 3 4
30. If you are disturbed by someone smoking near you, can you say so?. 0 1 2 3 4
31. Do you shout or use bullying tactics to get others to do as you wish?. 0 1 2 3 4
32. Do you finish other people's sentences for them?. 0 1 2 3 4
33. Do you get into physical fights with others, especially with strangers?. 0 1 2 3 4
34. At family meals, do you control the conversation?. 0 1 2 3 4
35. When you meet a stranger, are you the first to introduce yourself and begin a 0 1 2 3 4
    conversation?. . . . .

Now go back and circle the three statements that most often result in your giving up your powers and becoming passive or anger you so much you become aggressive.

3. Assertive, Aggressive and Passive Responses

Practice making responses to the following situations. The first situation is done for you as an example.

1. Saying no
   The head nurse stops you on the floor as you are just about to evaluate a new patient. "Mr. Johnson needs to be supervised in the use of his walker as he goes to the bathroom and none of us have time. I wonder if you'd mind walking with him right now."
   Passive—Well, I'm very busy, but if he has to go right now, I suppose I can help.
   Aggressive—Look, I taught him how to use that walker. It's your job to supervise him in bathroom activity. I've got a patient to evaluate, and I don't appreciate your inconsiderate views of the value of my time.
   Assertive—No, I can't do that right now. Mrs. Adams is able to help him, as can his family members. I have a new evaluation that can't wait.

2. Making requests
   It's the end of the day and you have three more patients to evaluate before leaving. You're going to need some help or you'll be working very late. How do you ask for it?

   Passive—

   Aggressive—

   Assertive—

3. Expressing opinions
   An edict comes down from above that *all* staff must teach a student for four to six weeks. You feel that you have too much to do already.

   Passive—

   Aggressive—

   Assertive—

4. Initiating conversation
You're attending a workshop and you've always wanted to talk with the speaker about a topic of great interest to you. You feel shy and somewhat intimidated by the speaker and her reputation.

Passive—

Aggressive—

Assertive—

5. Self-disclosing
Your parents are in the midst of a year-long divorce battle that has brought great grief to your younger brother. Last night he called you and spoke of thoughts of suicide. They live far away, and you feel frightened and helpless. At work, you seem distracted and upset. A friend asks, "Is there anything wrong? You seem preoccupied today."

Passive—

Aggressive—

Assertive—

6. Expressing affection
A patient that you have been working with is being discharged. You go to the room and his family is there packing to help him move back home. He asks to speak to you privately, and takes your hand and thanks you for everything you've done for him.

Passive—

Aggressive—

Assertive—

7. Entering a room of strangers
You've just moved to a new city to begin your first position after graduating. A new colleague invites you over for a party. You walk into the apartment and you realize you do not know one person in the room except the host. Everyone else seems to have known each other for years.

Passive—

Aggressive—

Assertive—

Reflect in your journal which of these situations was easiest for you to envision handling assertively, and which was most difficult. Which responses were easiest to come up with? Do you find that how you might respond has very much to do with your perception of the stress inherent in the situation?

4. The Male and Female Within Each of Us

Adapted from Gawain[11,p.52]

Carl Jung writes about the fact that each of us has both male and female energies inside of us. He termed these energies the anima (female) and the animus (male). Our task in living a balanced life is to develop these energies so that they can work in harmony with each other. Most of us have repressed one energy, and emphasized the other. The image of the strong, macho male is a caricature of a man who has no interest in exploring or developing his feminine, sensitive energy. The woman who dresses seductively and conveys the need for strong, masculine support in order to function at all is the extreme of the development of the anima at the expense of the animus. Most people in health care have had to develop a strong animus, which is our action energy, our ability to express the drive to succeed, in order to make it through rigorous health care curricula. Likewise, most people in health care have developed sensitivity to people in need (anima), or the health professions would hold little appeal.

The female energy within is the intuitive, creative energy, while the masculine energy within is the ability to act to get our goals and needs met. As they work together within us, we experience success and creativity. The female energy says, "I feel this," and the male energy responds with, "I hear you; this is what we can do about that feeling."[7]

This exercise invites you to explore your personal images of the masculine and feminine energies within you. Using deep breathing techniques, center yourself and quiet your dominant, overactive left brain.

Concentrate on your breathing for three minutes, remaining quiet and centered. Now bring to mind an image that represents your inner female. Look at her carefully; notice what she represents to you. Notice the details about her, the colors and textures. Ask her if she has anything she'd like to say to you.

Receive whatever she has to offer, be it words, images or feelings.

Now take a deep breath, and clear this image from your mind. Draw to mind an image that represents the male energy inside yourself. As before, notice the details about it. How do you feel about this energy? Ask him if he has anything he'd like to say to you.

Now ask both your male and female images to come to you at the same time. Watch them in relationship with each other. How do they relate? Ask them if they have anything they would like to say to you.

When you feel complete, take a deep breath and come back to the present. Journal about what you learned.

5. Assertive Communication

In this chapter you learned about DISC and DESC communication. Now you have a chance to role-play various assertive responses to the following vignettes. Before role-playing, however, you are asked to write the DISC or DESC response. The practitioner or student is in the assertive response position; the other person should use this opportunity to practice the active listening skills learned in the chapter just previous to this one. A third person serves as the observer, giving feedback at the end of the dialogue on the effectiveness of the communication. Use the Observer Response Sheet following Vignette 8 to jot down your observations as they occur. Each person should choose an appropriate "difficult" vignette, and write a DISC or DESC statement before breaking up into groups of 3.

Vignette 1

You are a student on your first of two final clinical assignments. The clinical facility is very high-powered with a superior reputation. You feel no matter what you do, you could never achieve the level that is expected of the staff. You truly feel that you're doing your best, but you are under constant stress to prove yourself. You are to be checked out on a knee evaluation, but you lack the basic skills, and you've asked for help from the star of the staff, who always says, "Yes, but I'm too busy. Catch me tomorrow." Your clinical instructor stops you as you are ready to go home and relax at the end of the day and says, "I've let you off the hook long enough. You should have that knee evaluation down by now. Come with me and let me check you out."

a) Write a DESC response
b) Role play

Vignette 2

You are a clinical instructor. You've observed your student for three weeks and feel he/she may be quite weak in evaluation skills, and you feel he/she is not taking the assignment seriously. When you suggest a checkoff session, your student always asks for more time. Yet all you hear is talk about lots of parties, after-hours fun, and you notice a real reluctance to read or show initiative in looking things up or asking for help. You think he/she might be trying to squeeze through without the appropriate amount of responsibility. You've decided to confront your student and ask for a checkoff on a knee evaluation.

Vignette 3

You've just accepted a position at a health care facility that also has an active student program. The staff seems to ignore the dress regulations and everyone wears what he or she wishes, and so you decide you will wear what you wish as well, and come to work in comfortable clothes with a lab coat, clearly not the dress regulation. Your supervisor tells you to go home and change your clothes and come back in the regulation uniform. You decide to confront him/her.

Vignette 4

In the middle of a treatment, your patient, a young and rather seductive member of the opposite sex, grabs your arm and tells you that he/she has very strong sexual feelings for you and wonders if you might meet privately at the end of the day.

Vignette 5

You are a professional on the staff for over a year. You still lack skill in one treatment technique that an aide knows how to do flawlessly. In front of the patient, the aide comes up to you and chastises you for not knowing how to do even the simplest procedures. You are embarrassed, and decide to confront the aide.

Vignette 6

Your colleague who always takes advantage of others comes up to you in front of a patient and asks you to cover for her, as she has to make an important phone call. She disappears and does not return for two hours.

Vignette 7

An older physician of the opposite sex is standing near you at the nursing station as you read your patient's chart. In front of his/her medical students, s/he winks at you and says, "Hi, Sweetie. Hurry up with my patient's chart, will you? I'm in a big hurry."

Vignette 8

Review your responses from the Assertiveness Inventory. Create a vignette that typifies a situation that is predictably problematic for you. Teach your partner how to act in a way that is sure to elicit passive or aggressive behavior from you. Then write a DISC or DESC response and role play.

Observer Response Sheet

As observer, your role is to facilitate a dialogue that has an adequate assertive response. The dialogue may begin with the "aggressor" making the statement that requires the assertive response, or it may begin with time having elapsed since the incident, and the assertive response is occurring now, some time since. Keep track of time, and keep the interchange to two or three minutes. At the conclusion, ask the assertive responder how he or she feels, then ask the other partner the same. Then proceed to give both feedback on the adequacy of their communication. How well did the assertive communicator:

1. Communicate using the "I" statements, DISC or DESC responses?

2. Stay nonaggressive, non-judgmental, nonaccusatory?

3. Listen and respond in an assertive way to the other's response?

4. How well did the "aggressor" use active listening skills and still stay in character? How would you suggest each could improve his/her communication?

chapter eight

THE HELPING INTERVIEW

Objectives

1. To emphasize the importance of communicating well in the initial stages of the relationship with the patient.
2. To describe the characteristics of a helping interview as compared to a nonhelping interview.
3. To teach the essentials of the helping interview.
4. To portray the qualities of a helpful interviewer.
5. To provide the opportunity to begin developing and practicing your interviewing skills.
6. To offer the opportunity to practice self critique and critique of others.

In this chapter we focus on another specific application of communication skill, the art of establishing the relationship with our patients and gleaning from them the information we need to be of most help to them. First impressions very often count, and the importance of obtaining the patient's trust from the outset of our interaction together is invaluable to the healing process.

Interviewing is much more than obtaining a patient history. The interview serves as the cornerstone for the structure of care we give. Patients come to us worried and often in pain. They feel vulnerable and in need of our help and understanding. They want, often desperately, to put this problem behind them and get on with their lives, and they know they can't do it by themselves. They come to us hoping that we will listen carefully, that we will know something about their problem, and will be able to help alleviate their worries; and they sincerely want to trust that they have made a wise decision in coming to us. Not only do they want physical and psychological comfort, they want another human being to resonate with their distress.[1] All of this emotion, in varying degrees of intensity depending on the patient and the problem, is presented to us upon our initial contact with the patient. Most people will utilize maximum coping skills, however, and few will fully reveal the extent of their feelings about their problem. Most adults will convey varying degrees of ability to remain in control in an environment that appears, at the least, strange and at the worst, hostile.

As health professionals, the burden is on us to recognize that the patient feels at a distinct disadvantage and to reassure and support even those who convey a remarkable sense of confidence and comfort. At this initial meeting, interest, genuineness, acceptance and positive regard are critical to establishing a healing relationship. And, as we have said before many times, the nature of the relationship we have with our patients is critical to the helping process.

Helpful Attitude and Skillful Questioning

Not only is it important to convey a healing attitude for our patients at the outset in the interview, it is imperative that the patient feel listened to and understood so that all of the information can surface that will lead to the most adequate and complete description of the problem. Thus, pragmatically, effective clinical decision-making depends on skillful interviewing. And skillful interviewing begins with a healing attitude and proceeds with artful questioning. Let's take a closer look at both.

The Healing Attitude of the Interview

A good interview depends on the appropriate attitude, good timing and artful phrasing.[2] The nature of the questions and the process of the interview session will flow out of the beliefs that the questioner holds about such things as one's self-esteem, the appropriate nature of one's role in healing, and what patients are like as people. Let's take a look at some ideas, beliefs and attitudes that facilitate a healing interview.

Positive self-esteem helps one assume a stance of "I'm OK and so are you. Neither of us is perfect, but each of us, I choose to believe, is doing the best we can to move forward in this world, and I want to help you get back to the business of life as soon as possible." This attitude fosters a healthy collegial relationship with the patient, and keeps the locus of control within the patient. Likewise, it hinders any tendency on the practitioner's part to lay blame on the patient for behavior that might have contributed to the problem he or she comes to us with.

A helpful belief of the nature of one's role in healing is to assist the person needing help to identify and cope with his or her problems quickly, and return to a feeling of being in control of one's life as soon as possible.

Patients are simply people who have a problem that they would solve by themselves, if they could. But they need our professional help to identify, clarify the nature and cause of the problem, and to help them solve their problem and get on with living.

Obstacles to Conveying a Healing Attitude

People who have an attitude that facilitates healing are able to accept their patients just as they are without judging them. These practitioners will often have identified and dealt with biases and prejudices about certain behaviors such as alcohol abuse, laziness, smoking, use of profanity, and obesity. They will have reconciled their abhorrence of some behaviors such as rape and murder and are willing to be therapeutically present to people accused of such behaviors. As much as possible, they will be aware of and willing to underplay and/or eliminates, deeply held prejudices about race, culture, gender, age or sexual orientation.

How does all this happen? Obviously not overnight. The paragraph above describes a mature person whose ego is not bound by the fear that emanates from immature judgmental and dualistic thinking. Behavior that is accepting is nonjudgmental or nonblaming in nature. As much as we might abhor a person's behavior, it is helpful to believe that the person would have acted differently if he had had more information and had been less impulsive.

Remember from Chapter Two that many of the immature judgments and prejudices we continue to carry as adults stem from fear that we developed as children from the messages we heard from adults around us. As adults, we must confront the inappropriateness and negativity of these judgments and work to establish more whole, accepting, self-affirming beliefs.

One of the purposes of this text is to assist you in this maturation process by helping you to identify harmful attitudes and behaviors that would interfere with the healing nature of the interview. Practicing our active listening skills and assertiveness skills helps in an interview. True active listening and speaking out of an awareness of your own rights help one to diminish a tendency to project one's own weaknesses and to minimize a judgmental attitude.

The Interview—Good Timing

With regard to timing, an effective interviewer avoids interruptions (which often reveals an underlying harmful attitude of "this person is not very important to me") and listens carefully, effectively using silence. Those who are uncomfortable with silence will miss much of what a person will say when given a chance to pause and reflect. Time is positively manipulated to indicate a seriousness of attention and level of involvement. A specific amount of time is set to spend, uninterrupted, listening to the patient carefully as he or she tells you the story of the problem.

The Interview—Artful Phrasing

Artful phrasing, a skill that is learned over time, involves using the right kind of question (open versus closed, direct versus indirect) at the right time, avoiding jargon, slang and dialect, and tuning one's words and gestures to reassure the patient that he or she is being attended to at a serious and thoughtful level.[2]

Stages of the Interview

There are three stages in the interview: initiation, or statement of the purpose of the interview, development or exploration, and closure.

The initiation of the interview takes place as you, the interviewer, explain who you are, why you are here, and the purpose of the interview.

The body of the interview is the development or exploration stage. In it the interviewer leads an exploration on the part of the patient, perhaps beginning with the open-ended question, "What brought you here today?" A good interviewer will guide the patient down a meaningful path, assisting the patient to explore his or her problem but not allowing the patient go too far afield from the problem. Active listening helps the patient to clarify and to zero in on the unique aspects of his or her situation. The interviewer listens carefully and sorts the information, jotting down significant revelations as he or she prepares for the clinical examination. The body of the interview unfolds in a unique story that the patient is invited and encouraged to tell. And the helpful interviewer confirms to the patient that he or she is being carefully and humanely listened to by a skilled and caring practitioner. When moving from one topic to another, it is helpful to use a transition statement. An example would be: "I think I understand the nature of your headaches; is it okay with you to shift now to the pain in your low back?"

The closing of the interview takes place at a time that has been predetermined by the interviewer. If it becomes obvious that the interview is not complete, the interviewer doesn't just let the session drop, but says, for example, "We're beginning to run out of time for this session and I realize you haven't yet finished. What needs to be covered yet?" Then a second session is scheduled. Or the interviewer may begin the physical examination, and continue discussing the problem with the patient during the exam. I offer a note of caution here, however; to begin the physical examination before allowing the patient to tell as complete a personal story as time allows is a mistake. As an interviewer, you cannot expect to establish a relationship and obtain meaningful information while engaging in palpation and physical evaluation methods. Your brain will attend to what you see and feel before it will attend to what it hears.

Body of the Interview—Information Gathered

The key questions that form the structure of the body of the interview, and that set the boundaries for a meaningful story from the patient include the following:

1. What is the patient's reason for seeking health care?
    Why did she or he come today?

2. What is the patient's perception of the problem? What is it? Why did it begin? What are the consequences of the problem?

3. What impact, if any, does the problem have on the patient's life? How does he or she feel about it? Does it affect work, relationships, quality of everyday life?

4. What are the characteristics of the problem?
   When did it begin? Precipitating factors?
   Where is it located?
   What is its quality and severity?
   What alleviates the problem?
   What makes it worse?
   What factors are associated with it?

5. What does the patient expect from this visit? What does he or she hope that you will do?

Use of Questions

Questions should be primarily open (exploratory), not closed (yes or no), and primarily indirect ("What do you think about. . .?") not direct (no discussion invited). You should avoid double questions (asking two questions at once), or bombarding the patient with several questions, forcing him or her to sort out what you're asking. The patient should be invited to ask questions, as well, and "why" questions should be rephrased to "what" questions to avoid a tendency to feel defensive. "Why" often seems to require a "because." "Why don't you rest in the afternoon when you feel pain?" can be rephrased to "What keeps you from resting in the afternoon when you feel pain?"

In sum, questions should be clear, open, indirect, encouraging reflection, single and nondefensive. Then you must listen carefully both to what is said and to what goes unsaid. You must listen with your intuition as well as your ears. And when you suspect a hidden or reluctant thought, gently suggest that you have a hunch that there's more that the patient hasn't said about that. Could that be so?

The active listening skills of restatement, reflection and clarification move the interview forward down a meaningful path. The patient should feel encouraged to tell his or her story, and feel assured that you believe he or she is capable of helping you to understand the problem. Patients will ask you for advice, and it is wise not to give it, but to help the patient decide what is best. Any overt or covert judgment, ridicule or disapproval will lower the patient's trust and stifle the flow of information and interfere with the quality of helping that can take place in the interview alone, even before you touch the patient physically.

Nonverbal Communication

The nonverbals communicated by the interviewer can either facilitate or hinder the quality of the interview. Key nonverbal elements of a helping interview include wise use of space (posture toward each other and at the same eye level, eliminating barriers), time (uninterrupted level of involvement), appropriate posture (leaning in, avoiding rigid posture or slouch or defiant gestures), voice inflection (appropriate speed and volume, warmth and genuine curiosity conveyed versus flatness or excessive use of "you know's"), eliminating of distracting body movements (twitching, shaking foot, tapping pencil), and good eye contact.

The Interview—A Unique Form of Communicating

Thus the interview represents a different form of communicating than we've learned growing up in our families and with our friends. The interview is the very first opportunity to convey a professional healing attitude, and it must be learned and practiced in order to develop skill. And behind every word needs to be an attitude of willingness and awareness that will result in congruence. The words and the inner attitude must be in harmony in order for the interview to be therapeutic. The interviewer must feel confident, peaceful, at one with self and genuinely willing to establish a healing relationship.

More on the Interview Attitude—What We Are

Alfred Benjamin[3] says,

When interviewing, we are left with what we are. We have no books then, no classroom lessons, no supporting person at our elbow. We are alone with the individual who has come to seek our help. How can we assist him (or her)? The same basic issues will confront us afresh whenever we face an interviewee for the first time. In summary they are:

1. Shall we allow ourselves to emerge as genuine human beings, or shall we hide behind our role, position, authority?

2. Shall we really try to listen with all our senses to the interviewee?

3. Shall we try to understand with him (her) empathically and acceptingly?

4. Shall we interpret his (her) behavior to him (her) in terms of his (her) frame of reference, our own, or society's?

5. Shall we evaluate his (her) thoughts, feelings, and actions and if so, in terms of whose values: his (hers), ours, or society's?

6. Shall we support, encourage, urge him (her) on, so that by leaning on us, hopefully he (she) may be able to rely on his (her) own strength one day?

7. Shall we question and probe, push and prod, causing him (her) to feel that we are in command and that once

all our queries have been answered, we shall provide the solutions he (she) is seeking?

8. Shall we guide him (her) in the direction we feel certain is the best for him (her)?

9. Shall we reject his (her),. . .thoughts and feelings, and insist that he (she) become like us, or at least conform to our perception of what he (she) should become?[3,p.156]

These are the central attitudinal questions that underlie every helping interview, and the response to each quite obviously reveals the values that form our attitudes. When you read the above questions carefully, you will see that Benjamin phrases a few to encourage a negative response, as if to have us examine our attitudes very carefully in order to be clear about our helping intentions. The humanistic values (and their subsequent actions) we discussed in previous chapters will lead to developing a healing attitude. Once that attitude is established, skillful and artful questions will become second nature, and the interview will become one more important tool in the practitioner's repertoire of healing behaviors. Automatically you will assume the proper listening posture, make sure that you are not interrupted, assume an active listening stance and convey a warm and genuine interest in your patient. And once this practiced routine becomes second nature, less stress will be attached to it, and you will experience great pleasure listening to most of your patients tell their story.

The Nonhelpful Interview

What would a nonhelpful interview look and sound like? Sometimes it is useful for us to explore a concept by describing its opposite. One interpretation of the opposite of a healing interview might go like this:

The clinician enters the treatment area where the patient has been waiting for quite awhile. Without looking up from the patient record, or acknowledging the patient in any way, the clinician begins to read the chart, and mumbles, "Mr. Zuck?"

The patient replies, "Yes," and the clinician continues to read.

Clinician: "So, what's wrong with you?"

Patient: "I'm not sure. I hurt my back. I can't work."

Clinician: No response but thinks to herself, "Oh no, another back. This is the third malingerer I have seen today."

Clinician: "Well, take off your shirt and climb up on the table."

She leaves the area and returns 10 minutes later and, without speaking, begins the physical examination.

This, as you can see, is not really an interview at all. No rapport has been established, no active listening done, no meaningful information is gathered. The practitioner values only the information she will get from her physical examination. The patient is reduced to a "thing," another "low back" in a parade of "low backs."

How would you feel if you were the patient? Would you, as many patients do, make excuses for the poor, overworked therapist whom you're grateful has made the time to see you? Or have you decided already that here is a person without manners who will treat you only as a thing, another event in a long and uninteresting day? Would you throw up your hands in frustration and bury your disappointment even one more time, further convinced that no one really cares about your pain, and that you must endure this alone, without the understanding help of another person?

Whatever "treatment" gets accomplished in the above example, it will be of far less quality than it could be had the clinician used helping interview skills.

Conclusion

If you have ever been fortunate enough to have observed a master clinician at work, you have seen a person who truly values the interview and devotes the kind of attention to it described in this chapter. The greatest obstacles to consistent use of the helping interview are overwork and burnout. The more we feel over-extended in our day, and the more we feel that we are repeatedly facing unresolvable problems, the more difficult it will be to come outside of ourselves with a therapeutic presence for the interview. Therefore, the very foundation of the helping interview is a commitment to the discipline required to keep a balance in our lives so that we're rested and have good energy to give to our work. Also, we are required to keep a reign on the extent we commit ourselves to the work that must be done, avoiding giving up the right to keep a reasonable pace. People who feel consistently overworked are avoiding the responsibility they have to keep control of the work load, and to fight for that right. Each patient we see ideally deserves 100% of our professional ability. It is our responsibility to make sure we have as much of ourselves to give as we can. Chapter Ten will expand on burnout, and help you learn to balance your lives so that this ideal is more reachable.

The exercises for this chapter, again, are critical to effective learning. Conducting a useful interview requires maturation, experience and practice. One of the most efficient ways to correct mistakes and improve style is to review videotapes of yourself interviewing in a role play and, if possible, with a patient. Maturation and experience lead to a quiet self-confidence and relaxation wherein the "third ear" automatically is engaged. Practice in interviewing will help you value and develop the artful balance of scientific discovery with compassionate intuition.

Don't forget to journal about this experience. What did you learn about yourself as an interviewer? What feelings did you have as you received feedback and/or watched yourself on videotape? Does a videotaping experience help you identify with patients even more than simply role playing? Again, have fun as you learn and grow and mature into the role of the healing professional.

References

1. Perlman, HH: *Relationship: The Heart of Helping People.* Chicago, University of Chicago Press.
2. Enelow, AJ and Swisher, SN: *Interviewing and Patient Care.* New York, Oxford University Press, 1972.
3. Benjamin, A: *The Helping Interview.* Second Edition. Boston, Houghton Mifflin, 1969.
4. Westberg, J and Schachner, T: Material from Interviewing Course in Health and Human Values, University of Miami School of Medicine, 1982-1988.

exercises

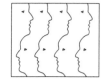

1. Responding to Situations

Below are situations in which you might likely find yourself as you interact with patients in the clinical setting. These situations are posed to help you explore in advance what you might feel in the situation, what may be underlying concerns in the situation, and what are some specific things you might say or do in a situation like this.[4]

1. You are scheduled to interview Dr. Reynolds and report your findings to your clinical supervisor. Dr. Reynolds has been waiting for you for over an hour, pacing up and down in the waiting area. When you go out to introduce yourself to her, she turns to you angrily and says, "You clinicians don't give a damn about other people's time. Do you realize how long I've been waiting out here?"

    How might you feel at this moment?

    What might the patient's underlying concerns include?

    What are some specific things you might say or do at this point to try to salvage the interview?

2. You walk into the patient's room, and he is watching television. You introduce yourself, and the patient never even takes his eyes off the TV. He acts as if you are not present in the room.

    How might you feel?

What might the patient's situation be?

What are some specific things you might say or do in this situation?

3. The person you are interviewing is a street person who has not bathed in a long time. She has a severe body odor, and an open sore on her leg that is infested with maggots. As she begins to speak to you, she asks for something to spit her tobacco into.

What might you feel?

What might be underlying the patient's behavior?

What might you say and do to insure a helping interview?

4. You begin an interview with Mr. Selker with a good, open-ended question, but soon after you begin he begins talking about his favorite football team. As you try to keep him on track about his problem, he consistently digresses to the topic of football.

How might you feel?

What may be underlying this patient's behavior?

What might you do to salvage the interview in the given amount of time allotted?

5. You are trying to conduct an interview with a patient, but each time you ask her a question, she looks to her husband, and he answers it for her.

What might you feel?

What might be underlying this situation?

What are some things you might say or do to get more information from the patient herself?

6. You are interviewing a patient about low back pain, and when you ask her how the pain is interfering with her life, she breaks down and sobs that she is no longer desired sexually by her husband.

What might you feel?

What might be underlying this situation?

What might you say or do at this point to maintain a helping quality to the interview? Practice your active listening skills of reflection and clarification.

7. You are interviewing a patient and the patient suddenly leans forward, grabs your arm and says, "You are so attractive. Are you married?"

What might you feel?

What might be underlying the patient's behavior?

What might you say or do to get the interview back on track?

8. You are interviewing an elderly patient who is sitting in a wheelchair. You believe he is able to understand you, but his responses are quite slow and labored. Suddenly you notice a stream of urine running down his leg and onto the floor. He seems not to pay attention to this.

What might you feel?

What decision must you make at this point of the interview?

What might you say or do to insure that the interview remains helpful in nature? Practice self-transposal. What would you want someone to say to you? To do?

2. Videotaping an Interview

This exercise is offered to help you develop skill in conducting the helping interview, and in critiquing your skills and the skills of your classmates. It consists of a role play of an interview which, ideally, should be videotaped. Each person in the class should have the opportunity to be taped. This may necessitate dividing the class into several small groups, each small group serving as an observation and feedback unit.

The exercise begins with each class member receiving a description of the patient he or she is to portray. This description should include all pertinent personal and illness (symptom) information so that the actor/actress can carry out the role completely. Completion of the *Patient Information Form* is important to this process. Students are to be invited to submit patient descriptions from their experiences, or simply make up a description of a patient's situation. Each student should complete a *Patient Information Form*.

Class members number off, but divide the class in half. If there are 50 students, number off 1 through 25, then start over and number 1 through 25 again. The two number 1's will interview each other. Each will role play his or her *own* patient described on the *Patient Information Form*.

Some rearranging may take place (for example, a woman student may prefer to interview another woman, or a man, whichever she feels she needs most practice with), but it is unwise to do much shifting around once the roles with numbers have been drawn.

When videotaping is done in small groups, an instructor should be with each group. The group should meet for as many sessions as it takes for each person to interview for 5 to 8 minutes. At that time the interview may not be over, but the instructor will call for an end.

During the interview, many thoughts and feelings are taking place. During the videotape playback, the interviewer has control of the pause button, and should stop the tape at any point he or she wishes to discuss the action and to review the various options that are available at that moment. The patient is invited to ask that the film be stopped as well, but the interviewer is in charge of the playback. Once the tape is stopped, the interviewer and the patient are invited to discuss thoughts and feelings, and classmates may feel free to question, emphasizing a noncritical curious attitude.

During the interview, observers are asked to complete the *Reviewer Assessment Form*. After the interview, the patient is asked to complete the *Patient Assessment Form*. During the discussion of the interview, reviewers may add comments on their assessment form. At the end of the entire process, the interviewer completes the *Interviewer's Self Critique Form*.

The total time for each interview session should take 20 to 30 minutes.

An Alternate Plan

Time and resource constraints may require that the patient and clinician meet outside class and arrange to have their interview videotaped, and then simply bring the tape to class for discussion and feedback. Classmates (reviewers) should have a summary description of the patient before viewing the tape, but, again, the class completes the *Reviewer Assessment Form* as they are watching the tape the first time.

Remember, the most important learning for this exercise grows out of the class discussion, not out of the tape itself. Feedback is best received when it is specific and given with kindness. Insights that contribute to learning are most effective when they are stimulated in a supportive and nonpunitive atmosphere.

You are reminded to journal about the experience. What was it like to play the role of an interviewer in front of a video camera and your classmates? What did you learn about yourself? What behaviors do you intend to develop?

Patient Information Form

Please answer the following questions about the situation which you will be representing in your role as a simulated patient. This exercise will be most useful if you answer each item as accurately, completely and authentically as a patient would who actually has the problem.

1. What is your reason for seeking care?

2. Why are you coming in to see the clinician *now*?

3. What other complaints or concerns have you had?

4. What do you think or fear the problem might be?

5. What do you think the consequences of the problem might be?

6. What are your past experiences with this problem?

7. How have your activities of daily living been modified as a result of this problem?

8. What other impact has this problem had on your life?

9. What has been the chronology of events in the development of this problem?

10. What is (are) the location(s) of the symptom(s)?

11. What is (are) quality(ies) of the symptom(s)?

12. What is (are) the quantity(ies) of the symptom(s) (i.e., frequency, duration, etc.)?

13. What factors have you noted aggravate or alleviate the problem?

14. In what setting does the problem seem to occur (e.g., what have you noted seems to precipitate the problem)?

15. What other manifestations or symptoms have you noted that seem to be associated with the problem?

16. What are your expectations of this visit to the therapist?

17. Describe your personal situation and characteristics.

18. What is the state of your underlying health?

19. What has been your past personal and medical history?

Adopted from Course in Health and Human Values; University of Miami School of Medicine, 1982-1985.

Reviewer Assessment Form

Circle the appropriate letters. KEY: Y = Yes; N = No; NA = Not Applicable
Note: Where indicated, use space under items to describe and give specific examples of what the Interviewer did.

Your Name _____

Interviewer's Name _____

Beginning of the Interview
Did he or she:

1. Greet the patient in a friendly, attentive, respectful manner?. . . . . .Y N NA

2. Attend to introductions of himself/herself and the patient, using the
   patient's name and his/her own name?. . . . . .Y N NA

3. Define the purpose of the interview?. . . . . .Y N NA

4. Help the patient get physically comfortable?. . . . . .Y N NA

Exploring the Patient's Concerns: Gathering Information
Did he or she: . . . .

4. Use questions appropriately?
   a. Use a "general open-ended approach" to help establish the
      reason(s) for the patient's visit?. . . . . .Y N NA
   b. Use a "topic oriented approach" to explore new topics; using
      specific questions only as needed? . . . . .Y N NA
   Give example:
   c. Avoid premature closed questions which can be answered "yes" or "no"?
      . . . . .Y N NA
   d. Ask one question at a time?. . . . . .Y N NA
   e. Refrain from using leading questions?. . . . . .Y N NA
   If used, give example:

5. Nonverbally communicate attentiveness and openness?. . . . . .Y N NA
   e.g., a. with a relaxed, open posture
         b. with facilitating gestures, like head nodding
         c. with natural, varied eye contact
   Describe:

6. Verbally communicate attentiveness and openness?. . . . . .Y N NA
   e.g., a. using encouraging phrases, like "Please, go on"?
         b. repeating key words or feelings
         c. "paraphrasing" reflecting back the essence of what the patient is saying
            and/or feeling
   Describe:

7. Remain silent, where appropriate?. .Y N NA
   e.g., a. give patient an adequate opportunity to questions
         b. didn't interrupt patient
   Describe:

8. Respond to patient in a warm and empathetic manner?. . . . . .Y N NA
   Describe:

9. Organize interview in orderly fashion?
   a. Proceed from the general to the specific?. . . . . .Y N NA
   b. Proceed from the less personal to the more personal?. . . . . .Y N NA
   c. In history taking proceed from present to past history?. . . . . . . .Y N NA
   d. When changing topics, make transitional statements?. . . . . .Y N NA
   Describe:

10. Speak clearly, using appropriate language without jargon?. . . . . .Y N NA

Closing the Interview (Complete only if Interviewer got this far.)
Did he or she:

11. Summarize what was said?. . . . . .Y N NA

12. Check if there were any further concerns or questions?. . . . . .Y N NA

13. Let patient know what will happen next?. . . . . .Y N NA

14. Other strategies Interviewer used which *facilitated* the interview.

15. Other strategies Interviewer used which *blocked* the interview.

Adopted from Course in Health and Human Values; University of Miami School of Medicine, 1982-1985.

Patient Assessment Form

Name of Patient:

Name of Interviewer:

In response to the following, please be as specific as possible.

Behaviors which facilitated my ability to communicate (e.g., your use of silence which gave me a chance to collect my thoughts).

Behaviors which blocked my ability to communicate (e.g., your use of leading questions, like "You don't have a sore throat, do you?").

Information and feelings, if any, that I was unable to share with you.

What I wished you had done or asked me.

Adopted from Course on Health and Human Values; University of Miami School of Medicine, 1982-1985.

Interviewer's Self Critique Form

Circle the appropriate letters: KEY: Y = Yes; N = No; NA = Not Applicable
   Note: Where indicated, use space under items and on back of document to describe and give specific examples of what you did.

Name _____ Date _____

Beginning of the Interview
Did I:

1. Greet the patient in a friendly, attentive, respectful manner?. . . . . .Y N NA
   2. Attend to introductions of myself and the patient, using the patient's name and my own
   name?. . . . . .Y N NA
3. Define the purpose of the interview?. . . . . .Y N NA
3a. Identify and reflect on my initial impressions of the patient. . . . . .Y N NA

Exploring the Patient's Concerns: Gathering Information
Did I:

4. Use questions appropriately?
   a. Use a "general open-ended approach" to help establish the reason(s) for the patient's visit.Y
   N   NA
   b. Use a "topic oriented approach" to explore new topics; using specific questions only as
   needed?. . . . . .Y N NA
   c. Avoid premature closed questions which can be answered "yes" or "no"?. . . .Y N NA
   d. Ask one question at a time?. . . . . .Y N NA
   e. Refrain from using leading questions?. .Y N NA
   If used, give example:

5. *Nonverbally* communicate attentiveness and openness? . . . . .Y N NA
   e.g., a. with a relaxed, open posture
         b. with facilitating gestures, like nodding my head
         c. with natural, varied eye contact
         Describe

6. *Verbally* communicate attentiveness and openness?. . . . . .Y N NA

7. Remain silent, where appropriate?. . . . . .Y N NA
   e.g., a. give patient an adequate opportunity to respond to questions.
         b. didn't interrupt patient
         Describe

8. Reflect on my own feelings and attitudes toward the patient?. . . . . .Y N NA
   Describe:

9. Organize interview in orderly fashion?
   a. Proceed from the general to the specific?. . . . . .Y N NA
   b. Proceed from the less personal to the more personal?. . . . . .Y N NA
   c. In history taking proceed from present to past history?. . . . . .Y N NA
   d. When changing topics, make transitional statements?. . . . . .Y N NA
   Describe:

10. Speak clearly, using appropriate language without jargon?. . . . . .Y N NA

Closing the Interview (Complete only if you got this far.)
Did I:

11. Summarize what was said?. . . . . .Y N NA

12. Check if there were any further concerns or questions?. . . . . .Y N NA

13. Let patient know what will happen next?. . . . . .Y N NA

14. Other strategies I used which *facilitated* the interview.

15. Other strategies which *blocked* the interview.

Adopted from Course on Health and Human Values; University of Miami School of Medicine, 1982-1985.

chapter nine

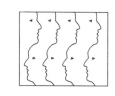

COMMUNICATING WITH THE DYING AND THEIR FAMILIES

Objectives

1. To clarify the importance of this topic to the maturation of the health professional.
2. To emphasize the importance of the therapeutic communication skills of touch and active listening.
3. To assist the reader to clarify current values around dying and death and to identify current comfort with the topic.
4. To delineate the knowledge and skill needed to facilitate a life of quality for the dying patient.
5. To describe the developmental stages health professionals go through as they learn to cope with the anxiety of caring for dying patients.

No one likes to contemplate death, except perhaps those for whom living has become entirely too painful. But to deny death totally throughout one's life, to refuse to reflect on the certainty that one day life will end for each one of us is to avoid a wonderful opportunity for enriching the quality of one's life. You've heard the phrase, "The unexamined life is not worth living." Elizabeth Kubler Ross has written:

> It is the denial of death that is partially responsible for people living empty, purposeless lives; for when you live as if you'll live

forever, it becomes too easy to postpone the things you know that you must do. You live your life in preparation for tomorrow or in remembrance of yesterday, and meanwhile, each today is lost. In contrast, when you fully understand that each day you awaken could be the last you have, you take the time that day to grow, to become more of who you really are to reach out to other human beings.[1]

Camus said, "There is only one liberty. . .to come to terms with death. After which, everything is possible."[2] Ernest Becker, in his Pulitzer prize winning book, *The Denial of Death*,[2] writes, "Of all the things that move men [and women], one of the principal ones is his [her] terror of death. . .All historical religions address themselves to this same problem of how to bear the end of life (pp. 11, 12)."

This may seem like an unlikely chapter for a book aimed at facilitating professional socialization, but I believe it deals with a topic that is most critical to the maturation of a health professional. To grow into one's profession requires personal growth along with professional growth. To deal with death greatly enhances this life task.

Some of you who have already lost a loved one will know what I mean when I say that this experience is unique in its ability to "grow one up" rapidly. James Agee, in *A Death in the Family*[3] recounts a tale of fresh grief as experienced by several members of one family following the sudden death of the husband and father in a car accident. Mary, wife of the victim, stands in front of a mirror ready to place the mourning veil over her face as she dresses for the funeral. She thinks to herself:

> I am carrying a heavier weight than I could have dreamed it possible for a human being to carry, yet I am living through it. . .She thought: this is simply what living is; I never realized before what it is. . .now I am more nearly a grown member of the human race; bearing children, which had seemed so much, was just so much apprenticeship. She thought that she had never before had a chance to realize the strength that human beings have to endure.

The Existential Fear of Death

Children are not born with a fear of death. At about age three, children begin to deal with object loss and experience both fear at the disappearance of the mother and joy at playing peek-a-boo. It isn't until age 10 or so that we begin to realize what it means for "life to disappear forever."[2,p.12] In fact, if fear of death were held constantly conscious, we would be unable to function normally. So we repress it, and by adulthood the common thought is, "I know I'll die one day, but I'm having too much fun living to worry about it."[2,p.17]

We can ignore our fears of death, or we can carefully absorb them and repress them in what Becker describes as our "life expanding process." With each victory in life comes a feeling of indestructibility, of proven power. Each time we notice the strength of our bodies, recover from the flu, avoid an automobile accident, or narrowly escape an injury or, more phenomenal yet, escape death, we further prove that we are indestructible. In addition, as we grow into secure and loving relationships with partners, parents and children, we feel secure support and appreciation for our existence, and a warmly enhanced sense of self acts to further repress the fear of our inevitable death. A healthy self-esteem doesn't have time to ponder death, we believe.

Only when death confronts us in remarkable ways do we even consider our own mortality. Besides near-death experiences, perhaps the deepest assault to our repression of the fear of death as health professionals is to care for a patient or a cherished family member who is close to the moment of death.

Why Concern Ourselves With Death and Dying in Health Care?

To come to terms with imminent death is one of the most difficult tasks human beings ever have to face, and we face it absolutely alone. No one can take our death away from us, nor give us the courage to die well. But the role others play at our side during this intense time can be either tremendously helpful or cruelly fragmenting and hurtful.

The quality of the help we render to those who are dying and their families has everything to do with our own ideas, values and fears about death, and until we clarify those ideas and values and confront our fears, we will be apt to increase the burden that is already almost too great to bear.

When death is imminent, we will be governed by what is deep inside of us, and our patients or loved ones will either benefit or suffer. If our fears of death predominate, we will deny the inevitable or defend fiercely against it. Out of our inner anxiety will emanate denial statements such as "Oh hogwash! You're healthier than I am! You're going to live forever!" or "Don't talk like that, Silly. It makes me depressed."

If our fears get stirred up too much, and our denial starts to break, we can expect anger and aggressive and passive aggressive assaults against those who are suffering. Just before we took my father home from the hospital to die (he was given six to eight weeks more to live after fighting cancer of the larynx with brain metastasis for the greater part of two years), the young nurse came to my father's hospital room and harshly asked, "Are you the daughter?" When I replied, "Yes, I'm John's daughter," he cautioned me as he flipped a vial of pills in front of my face, my father's medication for pain, "Now, don't give this to him when he asks for it; give it like the label says. I can't help it if he's in pain; he has to learn to endure it. If you give him medication every time he asks for it, and he comes back here to my unit, I'll have to be in his room every hour or so, and I have 30 other people who need me just as much as he does."

I felt frightened and assaulted in that moment by a person who had supposedly studied to be a healing professional. The more our behavior is governed by our denial and fear of death, the greater the chance that we will add to the already overwhelming burdens of the patient and the family as they struggle with one of life's deepest pains.

Author and dancer Isadora Duncan lost both her young children in a tragic accident in which a taxicab carrying them both fell in the water and they were drowned. After the accident, she fled to her friend, the Italian actress Eleanora Duse, at her villa in Italy. Her friend knew how to help her grieve and did not offer platitudes, or sit with her in embarrassed silence, offering her ideas and activities to "take her mind off her worries." She allowed Duncan to feel what had happened to her, to experience her loss. Duncan writes in *My Life:*[4]

> The next morning I drove out to see Duse. . .She took me in her arms and her wonderful eyes beamed upon me such love and tenderness that I felt just as Dante must have felt when, in 'Paradisio,' he encounters the Divine Beatrice.
>
> From then on I lived at Biareggio, finding courage from the radiance of Eleanora's eyes. She used to rock me in her arms, consoling my pain, but not only consoling me, for she seemed to take my sorrow to her own breast, and I realized that if I had not been able to bear the society of other people, it was because they all played the comedy of trying to cheer me with forgetfulness. Whereas Eleanora said:
>
> 'Tell me about Deidre and Patrick,' and made me repeat to her all their little sayings and ways, and show her their photos, which she kissed and cried over. She never said, 'Cease to grieve,' but she grieved with me, for the first time since their death, I felt I was not alone.

As a health professional, you will not be called to provide this level of support and caring. However, once people have matured and confronted their innate fears of death, we find that their ability to comfort and support the dying in whatever way is needed in the moment develops into quite profound skill and sensitivity. When we get beyond our defenses about death, we can then learn how to be therapeutically present for the dying. Life affirmation replaces death denial, and our actions are characterized by an intrinsic belief that life, moment to moment, is good and that we have the power to do something about the quality of a person's life, moment to moment. We realize that, even in the face of inevitable death, the support and comfort of family and mature healing professionals can actually help the patient transform his or her last days into some of the most rich and meaningful of his or her entire life. Confronting our fears of death is not easy, and we reflexively avoid it. But when we face this task with courage, we experience a quality of growth that is unparalleled in our development, personally and professionally.

Quality of Life is More Important than Quantity

Each one of us will die. We're only here for a short time on earth; that we know of. The average life expectancy of about 75 years may seem like forever to us, but as we approach that age, we will wonder where the years went. The lucky ones among us will have time to prepare for death. I believe this preparation time is a cherished gift, not just because it feels good to be able to tie up loose ends, to tell our dear friends how much life with them has meant to us, to make final arrangements, etc. In most cases, when you know your time is very limited, and you accept the inevitability of your death, the quality of that time increases exponentially. You become as liberated as a four-year-old in your intentions and in your communication. You ask for what you want, and you say what you really feel without the concern for whether someone will think ill of you, or not like you. This is a tremendously freeing experience. Commonly felt anxieties are replaced with living each moment just as you wish, for these are your last moments here on earth, and they are very precious, for few of us feel that we really know what lies beyond death. Genuine, heartfelt feelings are expressed. There is no time for superficialities or small talk, unless one chooses. Every conversation reflects deeply held thoughts and values. Great wisdom is passed along without fear of being accused of egocentrism. In fact, the predominant feeling becomes "What is to be feared now?" The ultimate fear has been confronted. The goal becomes how to live well the remaining time, rather than how to avoid death. This acceptance does not happen all at once, but takes place in stages over time, as I'll discuss in just a moment.

When we as health professionals take the opportunity to work with the dying, the quality of our lives can also improve. However, we find it far easier to be present to the dying who have accepted the inevitability of their imminent death, than to work with patients and families who refuse to face inevitable death, and live each day working furiously to maintain denial or controlling the anxiety of the inevitable. There are few worse situations in life than to try to be present in a therapeutic way to a patient or family who are denying imminent death. This situation most often develops out of a mistaken fear that the patient (or family) will lose hope, and the patient will give up the will to live. Studies reveal the opposite.[5] Depression and the loss of hope may appear as part of the coping of dealing with dying, but these feelings usually do not last long, and are replaced by hope for more realistic things. For example, patients will maintain their hope for a miracle all the while accepting the inevitability of death. Then, more pragmatically, they will shift their emphasis to, for example, the hope to live long enough to see a child be married, or to return home to see loved ones or pets.[5]

Stages of Loss

Elizabeth Kubler Ross, in her well known book, *On Death and Dying,*[5] describes what we can expect to experience as we go through the loss of a loved one, or experience our own dying. People initially experience a denial at the news of impending or actual death of a loved one. The most extreme forms of denial include total repression of the news or actually losing consciousness.

Denial is often followed by anger. Once we allow the news to begin to penetrate, intense feelings of anger can be expected to emerge. Health care workers must take care not to personalize this anger, but to allow patients to fully experience it and express it. This is made more difficult in a society that does not tolerate emotional outbursts of any kind.

Following anger, the patient often experiences a brief bargaining phase in which a kind of a deal is cut with life, or with fate, or God. For example, one will hear such thoughts as, "Okay, I know I'm going to die soon, but please let me live long enough to see my children get married." Or "If I can live, I'll never smoke another cigarette again."

Often the next stage that emerges is depression. Patients become quiet and more lethargic, reacting to the undeniability of this news as they live with it day after day. They keep to themselves, often refusing to see visitors or speak to certain family members. Reactive depression then leads into a preparatory depression in which patients quietly reflect on the sadness of their fate, and prepare for inevitable death.

Finally patients move into acceptance of their fate, and begin to live life as a precious gift. Not everyone reaches this stage before dying, and very often these stages do not occur in a linear sequence. It is quite common to hear a patient who seems to have worked through the stages into acceptance say, for example, "Next year I'm going to plant a different garden. I'm tired of the same old flowers. I'm going to rethink the whole layout and do it the way I always wanted to."

Thus the dynamics of coping with inevitable death take on a certain predictable rhythm and character, but each person copes in his or her unique way. Likewise, family members go through their own unique stage processes, and it can become quite complex just trying to keep track of where each person is in the process of accepting one person's imminent death. The patient may be in acceptance, but her husband may still be angry. Children may need to deny until the end. It takes great sensitivity and acceptance to be willing to be therapeutically present to each of these people, and requires that we choose to believe that each one is doing the very best he or she can, at the moment, to cope. It is not our role to force "reality" onto them.

Predictable Responses From Caregivers

Working with the dying can become a great challenge, depending on the extent to which we have confronted our own fears, and the extent to which

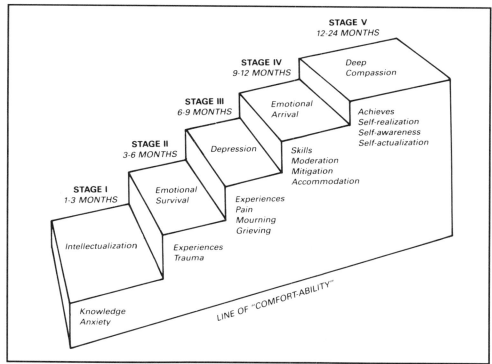

Figure 9-1. Coping with Professional Anxiety in Terminal Illness. Reprinted with permission from Harper, B: *Death, the Coping Mechanism of the Health Professional.* Greenville, SC, Southeastern University Press, Inc. 1977.

the patient and family have accepted the inevitability of the imminent death. What data exist to help us understand our natural responses to this caregiving challenge? How can we be guided to offer a healing response no matter what the atmosphere surrounding the patient?

Beatrice Harper has studied the development of health professionals' ability to cope with the anxiety surrounding the death of their patients.[6] Figures 9-1 and 9-2 illustrate the five stages of coping that she observed in social workers as they dealt with their anxiety about dying patients. She observed that the nature and intensity of anxiety of caregivers shifted in a developmentally predictable way from Stage One, Intellectualization, characterized by the need to deny and intellectualize death, to the inevitable Stage Five of Deep Compassion, characterized by the development of the ability to give of oneself and a feeling of comfort in relation to oneself, the patient, the family and the tasks of caregiving.

This figure can help you anticipate and analyze your responses when you first confront a patient who is dying. I offer it to assure you that your therapeutic skills in caring for the dying will develop and improve, and to remind you that caregiving for the terminally ill involves a personal as well as professional growth process. You should not expect yourself to be expert in this area from the very start.

STAGE I	STAGE II	STAGE III	STAGE IV	STAGE V
Professional Knowledge Intellectualization	Increasing Professional Knowledge Less Intellectualization	Deepening of Professional Knowledge Decreasing Intellectualization	Acceptance of Professional Knowledge Normal Intellectualization	Refining of Professional Knowledge Refining Intellectual Base
Anxiety Some Uncomfortableness	Emotional Survival Increasing Uncomfortableness	Depression Decreasing Uncomfortableness	Emotional Arrival Increasing Comfortableness	Deep Compassion Increased Comfortableness
Agreeableness Withdrawal	Guilt Frustration	Pain Mourning	Moderation Mitigation	Self-Realization Self-Awareness
Superficial Acceptance Providing Tangible Services	Sadness Initial Emotional Involvement	Grieving More Emotional Involvement	Accommodation Ego Mastery	Self-Actualization Professional Satisfaction
Utilization of Emotional Energy on Understanding the Setting Familiarizing Self With Policies and Procedures	Increasing Emotional Involvement Initial Understanding of the Magnitude of the Area of Practice	Over-Identification With the Patient Exploration of Own Feelings About Death	Coping With Loss of Relationship Freedom From Concern About Own Death	Acceptance of Death and Loss Rewarding Professional Growth and Development
Working With Families Rather Than Patients	Over-Identification With the Patient's Situation	Facing Own Death Coming to Grips With Feelings About Death	Developing Strong Ties With Dying Patients and Families Development of Ability to Work With, On Behalf of and for the Dying Patient	Development Ability to Give of One's Self Human and Professional Assessment
			Development of Professional Competence Productivity and Accomplishments	Constructive and Appropriate Activities Development of Feelings of Dignity and Self-Respect
			Healthy Interaction	Ability to Give Dignity and Self-Respect to Dying Patient Feeling of Comfortableness in Relation to Self, Patient, Family and the Job

Figure 9-2. Stage Characteristics and Differences of the Schematic Growth and Development Scale. Reprinted with permission from Harper, B: *Death, the Coping Mechanism of the Health Professional.* Greenville, SC, Southeastern University Press, Inc. 1977.

Therapeutic Presence in the Atmosphere of Denial of Imminent Death

The atmosphere of death denial is very uncomfortable. As was mentioned above, there seems to be an aura of fear surrounding the patient and family members; a false cheerfulness pervades that is edged with an iciness of the need to control every situation, every conversation. Instead of feelings of liberation, genuineness and authenticity, we feel surrounded by paranoia, fear, defensiveness, and nervous chatter. Silence is often avoided, as is warm eye contact.

When we contribute to the conspiracy of silence, we condemn a patient to the pain of facing death alone.[6] Our task is not to judge those who need to deny death, or to contribute to that conspiracy. Rather, we can help more by accepting their fear, and by realizing that their need to deny is very likely well-intentioned.

Active listening skills are imperative, as well as use of touch.[7] Health professionals would do well to find out what the patient has been told, and what the patient's response to what he or she has been told has been. Knowing what the patient has been told allows health professionals to support and interpret the health care team's plan of treatment. How the patient feels dictates the main thrust of the treatment approach.

Whether the patient has accepted the imminence of death or not, our approach to caring remains essentially the same. Debra Flomenhoft, a physical therapist who died of cancer, wrote the following important suggestions after having undergone treatment for over a year, in "Understanding and Helping People Who Have Cancer" published in *Physical Therapy*.[7]

1. Don't be afraid to say the wrong thing, and don't keep silent out of that fear. This is interpreted as avoidance and rejection. Instead of worrying about the content of your response, reach out to the patient and show your support by actively listening and allowing the patient to talk.

2. Learn to recognize your feelings and the effect these feelings may have on the communication process. Direct your predictable anger at something other than the patient.

3. When patients ask the hard questions, like, "Why me?" don't respond by trying to "fix it." Patients aren't looking for answers as much as they are expressing grief and anger. Allow that expression. Supportive listening is the best response.

4. Recognize the importance of touch, even as simple as a handshake or a touch on the shoulder. Communicate with touch and eye contact that you care, and that you are there to listen and to do whatever you can to maintain or improve the quality of the patient's life.

5. Don't assume that patients want to talk about their illness. Ask the patient if he or she wants to talk about his or her illness before initiating a discussion.

6. Never assume that you know what the patient is feeling. Ask instead, "Am I right that you are feeling. . .?"

7. Communicate confidence in your therapeutic skills both verbally and nonverbally. This is essential for patient trust. Answer the patient with authority and no hesitation, and if you don't know the answer, simply say, "I can't answer that, but I will find out who can."

8. Don't try to anticipate which stage of coping patients are in, or that they will progress through the stages in exact linear sequence. Accept patients where they are, each day, with caring and understanding. Try to view the impending death from the patient's perspective, not from the theory of dealing with loss.

9. Take care not to contribute to isolation of the patient as death nears. Once a relationship has been established, work to maintain it, even if the required therapy is minimal, or the patient has been discharged from your service. Stopping in to say hello, no matter how busy you are, will mean a great deal.

10. Help patients maintain hope at all costs. Maintaining hope is not in direct conflict with being realistic. The value of hope far exceeds the need to face the truth of the inevitable. One can feel hope in spite of imminent death, and it is important to nurture and sustain it, being both realistic and hopeful at the same time. Learn to communicate honestly and frankly, always with hope.

11. Take care of your own emotional needs to prevent professional burnout so that you can continue to communicate care, sympathy and support to the patient and family. If you need help in dealing with your feelings, get it. Your patient can't wait for you to grow at your own pace.[7]

What do dying patients want and deserve to have with regard to care? Figure 9-3 illustrates "The Dying Person's Bill of Rights," which was developed by the Southwestern Michigan Inservice Education Council.[12] Read each item carefully. They represent the minimal goals for care that we should all be guided by.

Hospice Care

One effective way of helping to assure therapeutic effectiveness in caring for the dying is the Hospice movement. Hospice is not a building, but a philosophy of care that promises that the patient will die with pain controlled to the greatest possible extent, and that the quality of life will become the primary focus of all treatment. Interdisciplinary team members each contrib-

---

THE DYING PERSON'S BILL OF RIGHTS

I have the right to be treated as a living human being until I die.

I have the right to maintain a sense of hopefulness, however changing its focus may be.

I have the right to be cared for by those who can maintain a sense of hopefulness, however changing this might be.

I have the right to express my feelings and emotions about my approaching death, in my own way.

I have the right to participate in decisions concerning my case.

I have the right to expect continuing medical and nursing attention even though "cure" goals must be changed to "comfort" goals.

I have the right not to die alone.

I have the right to be free from pain.

I have the right to have my questions answered honestly.

I have the right not to be deceived.

I have the right to have help from and for my family in accepting my death.

I have the right to die in peace and dignity.

I have the right to retain my individuality and not be judged for my decisions, which may be contrary to the beliefs of others.

I have the right to discuss and enlarge my religious and/or spiritual experiences, regardless of what they may mean to others.

I have the right to expect that the sanctity of the human body will be respected after death.

I have the right to be cared for by caring, sensitive, knowledgeable people who will attempt to understand my needs and will be able to gain some satisfaction in helping me face my death.

Used with permission: SE Mich. In Service Education Council Oakland Tribune, Oakland, CA (Sept. 30, 1978)

Figure 9-3. The Dying Person's Bill of Rights

---

ute to the care of the patient by direct services, often in the home, and by teaching family members and volunteers how to ensure that the quality of life for the patient remains as high as possible. Pain is controlled while maintaining alertness. Death is accepted as inevitable, and family members are encouraged to talk openly with patients in preparation for the time of death.

In addition to effective control of pain, it is important for the physical therapist to teach the patient and family how to keep the "lived world" of the patient as large as possible for as long as possible. By "lived world," I mean the world that is accessible to the patient to live in. Traditionally our lived world shrinks from almost limitless possibilities (given funds and opportunity to travel) to confinement to a chair or bed in one room as we age and become unable to move about. Range of motion, ambulation with support, bed mobility, getting up for meals, even placing the bed in the living room in front of a window all help to prevent the lived world of the patient from shrinking to a circle on the ceiling above the bed, as some patients have reported. The quality of life has every bit to do with how much of the world is available for us to experience.

Family members are encouraged to be around the patient as the patient requests. Pets are allowed to be close by. The atmosphere becomes one of living life fully.

Pain control is made possible through finely titrated narcotics, massage and exercise to the patient's tolerance and the use of TENS, or transcutaneous electrical stimulation to the nervous system. Data shows that patients respond very favorably to this modality, especially in the presence of severe, intractable pain often accompanying imminent death.[8]

Other Issues

This chapter does not have the space to deal with several important issues that accompany a consideration of death. The moral issues of "mercy killing" or euthanasia (both active and passive), suicide and the unique needs of persons with AIDS are just three issues that would require greater attention than this chapter can give them. After the fear of death is confronted, it becomes easier to read and study such topics independently. All are critically important to one's development as a healing professional.

Finally, there exists some controversy around the topic of near-death experiences as researched by Moody[13] and colleagues and around the person of Elizabeth Kubler-Ross.[14] Any consideration of death must, by necessity, border on the spiritual, for to ask, "Why have I lived?" is a spiritual question. It is within this category of awareness that much criticism is leveled at Kubler-Ross. I would encourage you to read about this controversy and form your own opinions. Once you have experienced the death of one who resides in your innermost circles of self, these readings, indeed, this entire chapter, will likely assume new meaning. For now, deal with this material seriously and as best you can.

Victor Frankl, a survivor of two Nazi death camps, has said, "Everything can be taken from a man [or woman] but one thing: the last of the human freedoms—to choose one's attitude in any given set of circumstances, to choose one's own way."[10] To accept death as a necessary part of life is not resignation; it is surrender to an opportunity to grow into one's own complete humanness.

I conclude with the following thoughts from Elizabeth Kubler-Ross:

> We are living in a time of uncertainty, anxiety, fear and despair. It is essential that you become aware of the light, power, and strength within each of you, and that you learn to use those inner resources in service of your own and others' growth. The world is in desperate need of human beings whose own level of growth is sufficient to enable them to learn to live and work with others cooperatively and lovingly, to care for others—not for what those others can do for you or for what they think of you, but rather in terms of what you can do for them. If you send forth love to others, you will receive in return the reflection of that love; because of your loving behavior, you will grow, and you will shine a light that will brighten the darkness of the time we live in—whether it is in a

sickroom of a dying patient, on the corner of a ghetto street in Harlem, or in your own home. Humankind will survive only through the commitment and involvement of individuals in their own and others' growth and development as human beings. [Through this commitment will come]. . .the evolution of the whole species to become all that humankind can and is meant to be. Death is the key to that evolution. For only when we understand the real meaning of death to human existence will we have the courage to become what we are destined to be.[1]

Conclusion

This text is devoted to helping you as health professionals grow to be mature and healing in your very nature, so that your actions with those needing your help will be healing and therapeutically whole. Elizabeth Kubler-Ross has said, "For only when we understand the real meaning of death to human existence will we have the courage to become what we are destined to be."[1]

The goals for this chapter, therefore, are for you to confront your own fears about death at whatever level you can at this time in order for you to become more aware of who you are to be. By way of reflection on this content and completing the exercises, you will conduct a current values clarification about death, remember your experiences of death as a younger person, and search for the blocks that would cause you to act in death-denying or angry ways rather than life-affirming ways.

What should our goals be with persons who are facing imminent death? In sum, what we want to achieve with the dying includes the following:

- assist the patient to remain in control of most decisions concerning daily life for as long as possible;
- keep the patient's "lived world" (the world available for the patient to move about in) as large as possible for as long as possible by helping the family learn to transfer or assist with ambulation or wheelchair management, assist with transfers out of bed, move the bed to an appropriate place to avoid isolation;
- control pain with medication, activity, imagery and TENS, yet allow maximum alertness;
- along with other health care team members, perform professional skills with self-confidence and patience, being sure to include the patient and family in the therapeutic process;
- provide support for loved ones and family, realizing each is in different stages of coping with the impending loss of a loved one;
- utilize active listening skills and touch as our primary forms of communication, allowing the dying person to have control over the topics and length of conversations;
- avoid the desire to want to "fix" anything;
- be willing to stand by, to touch, to reach out and to risk in the face of our own fears.

No easy task. Stanley Kellerman, in "Living Your Dying,[9] says, "There's big dying and there's little dying. . ." (p. 5). As health professionals we confront loss of health and mobility as a "little death" rather regularly. In your day-to-day patient care, always remember that people cope with little deaths similarly to big deaths.

So now move on to the exercises, and don't forget to journal about what you're feeling, and about what you've learned.

References

1. Kubler-Ross, E: *Death—The Final Stage of Growth.* Englewood Cliffs, New Jersey, Prentice Hall, Inc. 1975.
2. Becker, E: *The Denial of Death.* New York, The Free Press, 1973.
3. Agee, J: *A Death in the Family.* Grosset and Dunlap, Inc. 1957.
4. Duncan, I: *My Life.* Liveright Publishing Corporation, 1955.
5. Kubler Ross, E: *On Death and Dying.* New York, Macmillan, 1969.
6. Harper, B: *Death: The Coping Mechanisms of the Health Professional.* Greenville, S.C., Southeastern University Press Inc., 1977.
7. Flomenhoft, DA: Understanding and helping people who have cancer. *Physical Therapy,* 4:1232-1234, August, 1984.
8. Reuss, R: Hospice: One PT's personal account. *Clinical Management,* 4(6):28-37, American Physical Therapy Association.
9. Kellerman, S: *Living Your Dying.* New York, Random House, 1974.
10. Frankl, V: *Man's Search for Meaning.* New York, Washington Square Press, 1963.
11. Worden, JW, Proctor, W: *Personal Death Awareness.* Englewood Cliffs, New Jersey, Prentice Hall, Inc. 1976.
12. *Dying Person's Bill of Rights.* Southwestern Michigan Inservice Education Council.
13. Moody, R: The light beyond. *New Age Journal,* May-June 1988, pp. 55-67.
14. Nietzke, A: The miracle of Kubler-Ross. *Human Behavior Magazine,* 1977, pp. 206-211, 254.

exercises

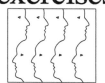

1. Personal Death History

Answer the following history questions below:

1. The first death I ever experienced was the death of:

2. I was   years old.

3. At that time I felt:

4. I was most curious about:

5. The things that frightened me most were:

6. The feelings I have now as I think of that death are:

7. The first funeral I ever attended was for:

8. The most intriguing thing about the funeral was:

9. I was most scared or upset at the funeral by:

10. The first personal acquaintance of my own age who died was:

11. I remember thinking:

12. I lost my first parent when I was:

13. The death of this parent was especially significant because:

14. The most recent death I experienced was when   died
     years ago.

15. The most traumatic death I ever experienced was:

16. At age   I personally came closest to death when:

17. The most significant loss I have ever had to endure was:
     because:

What insights come to you as you review your answers, or as you discuss your answers with a classmate? What do these answers have to do with your current ideas about death? The next exercise will help you clarify your current ideas.

Adopted from Worden and Proctor: Personal Death Awareness.[11]

2. Values Around Death and Dying

In order to better clarify your current feelings, attitudes and beliefs concerning death and dying, please reflect on and respond to the following questions:

1. When I die, I believe that: (what will happen?)

2. I would rather die: suddenly and without warning . . . or after being given a period of time in which to say goodbye to loved ones? What beliefs make me say this?

3. When I die, I'd like the following to be done. . .(be as specific as possible. Make a list.)

4. The person I want to be in charge of this process is:
   because:

5. The worst possible thing that could happen to me around my dying and death is:

6. As a health professional, the best thing I can do for my dying patients and their families is:
   because:

3. Life Line

Draw a line that best represents your total life span. At the end of the line, mark the year, and your age, at the point of your death. Indicate the up's and down's of your life by labeling them with words and dates.

Reflections: How does it feel to consider the total span of your life? Remember, feelings are one word, like anxious or exciting, not "I feel like my life. . ."

How would you characterize your life so far? More "up" than "down," or the reverse, or neutral? What are the major forces that have contributed to this assessment?

Do you have certain life goals that you can identify? If so, identify them, and then comment on how well you feel you are progressing toward them. Indicate what goals you expect to have achieved at certain points along your life line.

Journal about this experience.

chapter ten

STRESS MANAGEMENT
PREVENTING PROFESSIONAL BURNOUT

Objectives

1. To define burnout, and explore personal sources of stress.
2. To explore the effects of stress on the body and on our perceptions of situations.
3. To discuss the stress development model.
4. To describe external and internal factors that contribute to the build up of stress in professional helpers.
5. To explore mechanisms that interfere with the build-up of stress, and thus help us to control the negative effects of stress.

One of the most powerful rewards of the healing professions is the tremendous job satisfaction it brings. Most people enter the helping professions in order to work with people who need help in overcoming illness or disability, or to help well people stay well and fit. The expectation is that, here is a career in which I can assume that each day will be interesting and rewarding, and I can expect to feel a great deal of personal satisfaction and meaning in helping others. Few people ever anticipate, or prepare for the tremendous amount of stress that is inherent in the helping professions. Despite the deepest feelings of caring and altruism, caring for people who need help can bring with it great emotional and physical exhaustion to those who do not prepare for it.

Stress

Let's take a closer look at stress in general. Stress is a value neutral word, that is, it need not indicate something negative. In fact, stress is simply a response to being alive, and the human organism requires certain stress in order to have something to respond to, to live.

What we perceive as negative stress results from our inability to solve a problem or to reach a goal that is believed (or feared) to be unattainable. We feel out of control, and tension arises from attempts to figure out how to get back in control and reach our goal.[1] It's like standing at the bottom of a huge mountain, and not knowing how in the world we'll ever manage to get to the top.

This kind of stress has effects on our perspective of the situation, and it has effects on our bodies. When we feel the anxiety of negative stress, we tend to misread the situation at hand, we tend to blow things out of proportion, take on unrealistic guilt or internalize and personalize thoughts that have little to do with us.[1] For example, let's say you feel under the stress of seeing five more patients in the next 15 minutes (an unattainable goal) and a colleague comes into your office and is noticeably upset about something. There's a high likelihood that one of your immediate responses to your colleague would be, "Oh great! What did *I do now*?"

The fact is that often you are not the cause of another person's anger or frustration, and you increase your stress by making that erroneous assumption. Under stress you've simply distorted a situation and, depending on the energy of your paranoia, blown it all out of proportion. Stress distorts our ability to see the world as it truly is, and this distortion then increases our stress, causing a positive progression or escalation of our anxiety. The greater the existing stress, the more likely the addition of more stress. In other words, a positive feedback loop is established.

Stressors Commonly Experienced by Students

Purtilo discusses ongoing anxieties commonly related to student life.[1] Remember that negative stress is experienced in the presence of a fear that a goal that we've set is unattainable. She reports that students respond most dramatically to three anxiety-provoking questions throughout their education:

1. Am I good enough?
   Not only troublesome just before exams, but an ongoing fear related to questions of moral and intellectual competence—in other words, this is an issue of self-esteem and can be fueled by constant comparison of oneself to "more talented" classmates and professionals.

2. Do I have what it takes?

   Similar to question one, this relates to perceptions of and fears about one's physical and emotional limits. This anxiety rears its ugly head the first time a student feels faint while in a hospital, or experiences the exhaustion of long hours of work without breaks.

3. Can I pay?

   The cost of tuition is steadily rising without a concurrent increase in financial aid. The anxiety of having to take out another loan, take on another job, or quit altogether weighs on students and often affects their performance in classes and clinics.

Life issues go on while students are in school, and as the age of students entering the professions increases, life issues become more complex, with families and partners to be concerned about. For example, illnesses, pregnancies, having to move, and marital and/or parent problems don't automatically disappear while the student finishes his or her education. These anxieties feed into the base level of life stress and can markedly affect students' abilities to learn.

Physical Effects of Stress

Stress takes its toll physically, as well. Now that medicine has made great strides in eradicating infectious disease, most illnesses are of a chronic nature, and most chronic diseases have been found to be greatly influenced by stress. When we perceive stress, the endocrine system goes into action. This was quite useful when we depended upon the sympathetic nervous system for our survival in the jungle. "Fight or flight" was at one time our only alternative in stressful situations, most of which were, indeed, life-threatening. However, it seems as if our nervous system has not kept up with our progress as a civilized society. Few wild animals threaten our survival, but in some situations we respond as if that were exactly the case.[2] This outpouring of adrenalin and other neuropeptides[3] acts as a stressor on our bodies. People's physical responses differ. Some suffer from headaches, others from diarrhea, nausea, cardiac palpitations, etc. Over time, organ systems break down under this constant stress and the result might be diabetes, high blood pressure, ulcers, colitis or arthritis, or chronic fatigue.

Stress Development Model

The key to understanding stress and preventing its negative effects lies in understanding the following model:

Life situation → Perception → Emotion → Physiological Response → Disease

The life situation is not the key component in this model; it is the perception that I have that this life situation is a tiger that is going to eat me unless I get out of here fast, or fight like crazy for my survival. Some people live all day every day as if there were a tiger just around the corner. They've learned a world view that life is a hostile place and one must always be on guard.[2] (Remember that Chapter Two gives us insights into how people learn this world view.) Others of us simply periodically find ourselves in situations where we realize that our stress is too high, and that our world view has been distorted and it's time to get a grip on things here, time to do what we must to get back in control of our lives.

How Misperceptions Develop

When there is, indeed, a misperception of the current situation, it is most often a result of the influence of past experience. We become programmed, in a sense, based on unfortunate things that have happened to us in the past, and thus we misperceive what is happening right now and we fear the unknown of the future. As a result, we allow history or old data to distort the present, and our anxiety mounts.

The key, then, to changing the negative effects of stress is to examine carefully our misperceptions. If we can interrupt the stress build-up by changing what we believe about what is happening, then the emotion will be more realistic, and the sympathetic nervous system need not be over-stimulated.

Learning to "stay in the present" is a place to start. As soon as we begin to feel anxious, we should take a deep breath and simply say to ourselves, "Stay in the now. Do not be influenced by the past that is gone forever, or the future that has yet to happen. Listen carefully to what is going on now. Do not personalize or react. Listen."[2] This is not an easy thing to do, for our reactions are firmly set in place by years of habitual ways of thinking. To interrupt these ingrained habits takes conscious practice and commitment to change. The skill of staying in the "now" is best learned by purposefully quieting your mind. This can be done by learning meditation techniques such as Transcendental Meditation,[3] or by practicing tracking your breath for 10-30 minutes every day. Sit quietly and practice focusing 100% of your concentration on the breath as it flows in and out of your nostrils. Quiet the "monkey-chatter" in your brain, let all thoughts float away in imaginary bubbles, and simply breathe. Soon your body will relax, and your endocrine system will help you to slow down and feel more centered and peaceful.

Burnout

Burnout is a term that has been popularized to indicate a state of emotional and physical exhaustion that results from intense and long-standing professional stress. Christina Maslach first described burnout in 1976.[4] Interestingly, the subjects in her investigation were human service personnel, or people helpers. The fact is that when we agree to help people, there are always professional demands that seem impossible to meet, and this creates stress and tension that builds over time. This professional stress and tension has been termed "burnout," and it is a dynamic process that is fed by a negative self-concept and negative job attitudes, which result in a loss of concern for people, a withdrawal from interaction, and alienation from the work environment.[5]

Signs and Symptoms of Burnout

Health professionals enter the professions with enthusiasm and optimism, and often soon realize that the demands of the work far exceed their expectations. The common response is to double the effort, with little change in productivity.[5] Soon fatigue and discouragement set in.

The stress of the intense emotional demands of health care interaction builds, and a common coping mechanism is to distance oneself, or become emotionally detached from work.[5] Detachment is often unconscious and can take the form of actual physical withdrawal, spending shorter time with people, or emotional withdrawal, objectifying people, for example, by labeling them. A patient with back pain becomes "the low back in 343."

Other signs of burnout are the drawing of crisp boundaries between work and home, compartmentalizing one's life sharply; and demonstrating less creativity in treatment, offering more rigid, "by the book" responses to problems, lowering the risk of making a mistake. Feelings of personal inadequacy from not achieving (often unrealistic) goals can result in self dissatisfaction which results in projected anger and frustration. People tend to stay away from you because of your "short fuse."

At home burnout can contribute to marital tension. There is a tendency to engage in compulsive behavior (addictions) to numb oneself from stress, so use of food, drugs, sex, and alcohol may increase. Physical signs such as headaches, stomach ailments, problems with elimination begin to appear. Sleep may be disturbed. By this time one is well on the way to increased absenteeism and begins to job hunt or seriously considers applying to graduate school, often believing that finding the right "place" to work, or be, will solve all of these problems.

Table 10-1 illustrates that the symptoms of burnout permeate several areas of our lives and build over time, and, as they escalate, they can be seen to fall into four stages. Stage One, Enthusiasm, characterizes the symptoms of early burnout mentioned before. Without appropriate intervention, a person inevitably progresses to Stage Four which carries many of the symptoms of a full scale depression.[6] Stage Four burnout is a serious condition, and very often professional help is needed to free oneself from this situation.

Table 10–1.

Manifestations of burnout in occupational therapists.

Components	Stage 1: Enthusiasm	Stage 2: Stagnation	Stage 3: Frustration	Stage 4: Apathy
Personal characteristics	Do I invest my whole self in my work?	Am I beginning to question whether I like my job and whether it meets my personal needs?	Am I not only questioning the value of my job but also the value of the entire profession?	Am I feeling totally disinterested in my job?
	Do I set extremely high goals for myself?	Am I beginning to see that there are limitations in my work environment?	Do I blame myself when a patient does not improve or return to treatment?	Do I avoid work by using all of my sick time? Am I disinterested in patient progress?
Modality use	Do I work toward increasing my repertoire of activities and/or attempt to create new program ideas?	Do I find myself using the same activities over and over again?	Is my stress so great that I no longer feel creative?	Do I always let the patients choose their activity, even when another modality may be more therapeutic?
	Do I verbally discuss with my patients the purpose of an activity and the progress that I have observed?	Do I focus with the patient on only one or two aspects of their performance?	Do I look at product versus process?	Am I disinterested in my patient's response to the modality selected?
Use of theoretical base	Am I interested in learning about new theories and applying them to my practice?	Do I prefer to use the theory base with which I am most comfortable? Do I attempt to use new concepts after discussion with peers and supervisors?	Do I find new theories to be a waste of time and mere professional jargon?	Do I find myself using no theoretical base at all?

Table 10–1. (continued)

Components	Stage 1: Enthusiasm	Stage 2: Stagnation	Stage 3: Frustration	Stage 4: Apathy
Interdisciplinary relationships	Do I attempt to engage other disciplines in the activity process? Do I work to increase communication among team members and to effectively resolve conflicts?	Do I get annoyed when people from other disciplines ask to observe my groups? Do I feel that my domain is being stepped on by other team members?	Do I feel competitive with other team members and avoid talking to them outside required meetings? Do I find myself expressing my anger about the team to the other therapists in my department?	Do I feel there is no need to deal with my team about unresolved issues because nothing helps?
Education	Do I enjoy the opportunity to educate others about what I do as an occupational therapist?	Do I get tired of always having to explain my practice?	Am I beginning to represent the need to always educate others, especially team members?	Do I avoid having to explain what to do?
Budget	Do I find it easy to adapt to a low budget by finding creative ways to use limited supplies?	Am I becoming tired of the constant need to adapt my programs to supply and budget constraints?	Do I find myself frequently complaining to my coworkers and supervisor about our limited budget and supplies?	Have I given in to our low budget by limiting my program to only those supplies that are readily available?
Response to supervision and increased responsibilities	Do I look forward to supervision and the opportunity to improve my job performance?	Do I become anxious when my supervisor suggests a change or that I take on additional responsibilities?	Do I resent changes implemented within the department and frequently discuss my resentment with my peers?	Do I avoid work because of what will happen next?
Professional development	Do I actively pursue workshops, seminars, and courses to improve my skills? Do I put a lot of energy into my professional organizations?	Do I find that outside of work I always choose to pursue activities other than continuing education? Am I questioning the value of the profession and its organization?	Do I find suggestions to pursue continuing education to be an imposition? Will I pursue these activities only on work time?	Am I disinterested in professional activities and continuing education?

Reprinted with permission from Apter LC, Kolodner EL:Professional burnout—are you a candidate? *Phys Ther Forum* 1987;6:10.

Causes of Burnout

Factors that lead to burnout can be grouped into internal and external causes.

External causes include conditions in the workplace that make it virtually impossible to experience consistent success such as:

1. Work overload
    — Understaffed conditions.
    — Overload of too many of one type of patient or one type of activity; not enough variety.
    — Inability to use professional skills and creativity due to lack of time.

2. Role ambiguity
    — Less than clear guidelines of boundaries of responsibility.
    — Nebulous expectations not communicated clearly.

3. Role conflict
    — Several professionals perceive they are responsible for achieving the same goal. Especially apparent in multidisciplinary team situations in which there is inadequate communication.
    — Physicians make all decisions with no regard for input from other professionals.[5]

Internal causes of burnout are more difficult to identify and often are more challenging to influence. They include:

1. Professional's self-esteem.
    How individuals view themselves personally and professionally has impact on their work. Low self-esteem facilitates imagined feelings of failure.

2. Inability to set clear boundaries between personal and professional needs.
    Unclear ideas about the motives for wanting to help people (i.e., the desire to "fix it" for people rather than encouraging autonomy) results in inadvertently contributing to patients' neediness and dependence on health care workers, which results in a feeling of becoming too close, or trapped in a relationship with a patient.

3. The establishment of unrealistically optimistic goals for patients and the failure to meet them, which lowers self-image.
    A common event from overachieving new graduates. Intervention and guidance is required from mentors or supervisors.[5]

Intervention

Previously we've discussed the importance of perception in handling stress. Cultivating an ability to "stay present" or "stay in the now," resisting the habit of interpreting present, ongoing events from past history, or fear of the future will greatly assist one to remain clear and realistic from moment to moment. Asking clarification questions and employing active listening skills will reduce the tendency to personalize and take undue responsibility for others' problems.

But the next step in reducing the problem of burnout is recognition that it is occurring, that it is happening right now to you, and choosing to believe that you have the power to stop its escalation. Since burnout has both internal and external antecedents, intervention must take place in both areas.[5]

Externally or organizationally, lowering staff-patient ratios is critical as is allowing for time away from contact with patients. Time doing less stressful work, such as record-keeping, reading journal articles, planning patient research, student education or quality assurance activity are effective ways to lower the stress exacerbated by intense interaction with people.[4]

Required use of vacation time also helps those who tend to overwork and deny the presence of burnout.[5] Mixing of patient loads and scheduling of regular staff rotations also help reduce the stress of seeing too many of one type of patient.[5]

Organizationally sanctioned support groups are also an effective way to help reduce stress.[9] In these sessions, discussion of feelings is more important than discussion of patient problems.[7] Many health professionals keep fears and feelings of personal failure to themselves, but most will welcome the opportunity to discuss frustrations concerning patients, especially if the organization encourages this opportunity for all its members.[7]

In rehabilitation we must maintain a constant awareness that strict adherence to the medical model of diagnose, treat, discharge "cured" very often does not apply to our patients. Most patients we see have multiple chronic illnesses and we must learn how to expect an appropriate amount of effort from them, maintaining a somewhat more realistic goal than a hope for a cure.[5] Patients' values and hopes must be clearly delineated and integrated into any plan of care.[8]

Studying burnout and its prevention while still in school gives you an added advantage before you get caught up in the confusing situations that your first position offers. Internally, or personally, health care professionals must develop a realistic view of helping and learn effective ways to handle repeated, intense, emotional interactions with people.[5] Regular exercise is critical in reducing stress. A lunch break that is taken away from the patient care milieu and that includes a brisk walk, bike ride or swim has immediate and long-term positive benefits. Sufficient sleep and a nutritional diet also serve to keep one's internal stress low.

The logical, systematic left brain is the seat of the anxiety that leads to burnout. It is the left brain that can't seem to figure out how to get the goal met. The right brain, however, is the source of relief from this pressure. The right brain functions by way of pictures, symbols, colors and dreams.

Meditation and activities that balance left and right brain activity and engage the right brain in activities such as daydreaming or imagery for relaxation during breaks in the work day also help.[8] Tracking your breath, as described earlier, is one such activity.

Above and beyond all, however, is the importance of each health professional carefully examining his or her own needs in becoming a health care worker in order to identify and curtail the tendency to overwork that is so common among us.[5] Workaholism is an addiction just as is alcohol or food or drugs. We engage in compulsive behavior in order to keep from dealing with our problems or from feeling the pain of normal growth and development. When work is used to keep us from growing, everyone suffers. Unfortunately, unlike drugs and alcohol that do not carry public sanction, workaholics are often praised for their dedication, and allow themselves to be taken advantage of by others.

Eventually workaholics come to the realization that they are receiving from their efforts far less than they are contributing, and often this awareness leads to a temporary decrease in activity. But unless the original pain and need for personal growth are examined and confronted at this time, a new addictive behavior will move in rapidly to fill the void. Remember that Chapter Two focuses on the need to not only confront compulsive behavior, but to locate and communicate with the abandoned child within all of us to begin the healing process before real change can be experienced.

Prevention

Since stress occurs from the perception of the inability to successfully achieve goals, one way to prevent this from occurring is to set goals that are predictably attainable. Stewart writes, "Unless the goals of therapy are agreed upon in the beginning, the therapist and the patient can be forced to work together over a long period of time attempting to achieve goals which are not shared by both."[9] When working with patients, Stewart suggests the following steps to help lower stress:

1. Establish a clear contract with the patient. This should contain an explicit description of the goals and responsibilities of both parties, and should take into account the patients' values and priorities.

2. Do not promise more than you are prepared to deliver to the patient, the family or referring practitioner.

3. Be aware of the patient's feelings of dependency, loneliness, and fears of abandonment. Deal with feelings with active listening, encouraging open discussion. Give plenty of advance notice before taking time off or separating from patients in any way.

Another skill that is useful in helping to keep control over the work environment is assertiveness training, for those who lack the skills needed to communicate ideas for change. Learning how to speak up from a position of personal confidence can help revitalize an entire work setting.[8]

Conclusion

Health professionals are responsible for clearly understanding the patient's problem, using a wide range of skills and knowledge to treat the problem, and, perhaps most important and most stressful, we are responsible for teaching the patient how to avoid future problems; we are responsible for helping people take responsibility for themselves and their health. This can be the most demanding of our obligations to those we serve. We must learn to handle situations that fail to respond to our interventions. We must learn to set realistic limits as to what we're willing and able to do to facilitate change. We must learn to face the inevitability of terminal illness and death. Each of these realities in health care, if perceived as failure, will cause stress, as the ideal, hoped for goal of cure and wellness is unattainable. We set ourselves up to experience burnout if curing is our only goal in health care.

When one enters the health professions, there must be an early commitment to taking care of oneself in order to prevent the negative effects of inevitable stress. In a previous chapter we discussed that people can be seen to be composed of four quadrants: the physical, the intellectual, the emotional and the spiritual. To avoid stress, one must keep a healthy balance of activity and growth in all four quadrants. This would include a commitment to eat well, get enough rest and sleep, get regular exercise, time away from people, emotional confirmation and support, and dedication to play and fun. Many of us who become health professionals who grew up in troubled homes have had to be serious from the very start, and we lack the ability for spontaneous play. If that is true, we must find others to help us. Our healthy survival depends on it.

The exercises are designed to help you identify the amount of stress you are currently experiencing and how that stress affects you physically.

References

1. Purtilo, RB: *Health Professional/Patient Interaction.* Third Edition. Philadelphia, W.B. Saunders, 1982.
2. Keyes, K: *Handbook to Higher Consciousness.* Coos Bay, Oregon, Living Love Publications, 1975.
3. Chopra, D: *Ageless Body, Timeless Mind: The Quantum Alternative to Growing Old.* New York, NY: Harmony Books, 1993.
4. Maslach, C: Burned-out. *Human Behavior.* 5:16-22, 1976.
5. Wolfe, GA: Burnout of therapists inevitable or preventable? *Phys Ther* 61:1046-1050, 1981.
6. Apter, LC, Kolodner, EL: Professional burnout—are you a candidate? *Phys Ther Forum* 6:6, 10, 1987.
7. Pines, A, Maslach, C: Characteristics of staff burnout in mental health settings. *Hosp Community Psychiatry* 29:233-237, 1978.
8. Davis, CM: The "difficult" elderly patient: stressful effects on the therapist. *Topics in Geriatric Rehabilitation* 3:74-84, April, 1988.
9. Stewart, TD: Psychotherapy and physical therapy common grounds. *Phys Ther* 57:279-283, 1977.

exercises

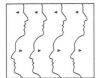

1. Recognizing Professional Stress

I realize I am stressed when:

which makes me feel:

and react by:

Afterwards, thinking about it calmly and quietly, I realize and tell myself next time I may choose to:

Signs and symptoms of burnout for *me*:

1.

2.

3.

4.

5.

Coping mechanisms which I use now within my environment:

1.

2.

3.

4.

5.

Three things I did last week to take care of myself:

1.

2.

3.

2. Holmes Stress Quotient Inventory

The emphasis in this chapter has been on revealing the effects of negative stress on the body and on the emotions. Hans Selye has identified that both positive and negative stressors affect people. Thomas Holmes has published research that correlates the effects of both positive and negative stress. Certain stressors are given a relative value or quotient with regard to their potential effects. Complete the following Holmes Stress Quotient Inventory. How vulnerable are you to the effects of stress at this point in time?

3. Physical Stress Symptom Scale

In most families, people react to stress in similar ways. The data is inconclusive as to whether this is primarily due to genetic weakness or learned behavior, but it is common to see several people in a family respond to stress with similar symptoms. The following Physical Stress Symptom Scale will help you identify which organs or systems are most vulnerable to stress. You may want to compare your results with other members of your family.

4. Major Sources of Stress in Students

Purtilo mentions that there are three major sources of anxiety for students[1]:
1. Am I good enough? (basically)
2. Do I have what it takes? (physically, emotionally)
3. Can I pay?

First of all, do you agree that these are stressors for you? What would you add to that list? Are there life issues that cause you stress, for example, developing identity and finding a life partner? Is the task of breaking away from your home and parents a major stress for you? Are you concerned that you may have chosen the wrong profession? Do you have a habit of procrastinating that gets you into trouble rather consistently? Make a personal list of stressors and prioritize them. Assign relative stress points to each item. Now journal about how those stressors affect you each day physically, emotionally, mentally and spiritually. For each stressor, list any actions you might be able and willing to take right now to minimize their negative effects. Finally, write about what you must simply surrender to time or fate or the universe, and learn to put away anxiety about things you have no control over. Carrying a list of constant worries around in your mind or on your back makes it difficult to be present to the world and to people. Develop the habit of taking a regular inventory of what you're worried about, what you can do about it right now, and what you must "offer up" and get off your mind. Make it a goal regularly to flush your mind and your heart of anxieties that are not appropriate or welcome. You'll feel lighter if you do.

Measure Your Stress Quotient

This stress rating chart, designed by Dr. Thomas H. Holmes, provides a measurement of the stress in your life. Check the events that have happened to you in the past year and then add up the total.

EVENT	VALUE
Death of Spouse	100
Divorce	73
Marital Separation	65
Jail Term	63
Death of Close Family Member	63
Personal Injury or Illness	53
Marriage	50
Fired from Work	47
Marital Reconciliation	45
Retirement	45
Change in Family Member's Health	44
Pregnancy	40
Sex Difficulties	39
Addition to Family	39
Business Readjustment	39
Change in Number of Marital Arguments	35
Mortgage or Loan over $10,000	31
Foreclosure of Mortgage or Loan	30
Change in Work Responsibilities	29
Son or Daughter Leaving Home	29
Change in Financial Status	38
Death of Close Friend	37
Change to Different Line of Work	36
Trouble with In-Laws	29
Outstanding Personal Achievement	28
Spouse Begins or Stops Work	26
Starting or Finishing School	26
Change in Living Conditions	25
Revision of Personal Habits	24
Trouble with Boss	23
Change in Work Hours, Conditions	20
Change in Residence	20
Change in Schools	20
Change in Church Activities	19
Change in Social Activities	18
Mortgage or Loan Under $10,000	17
Change in Sleeping Habits	16
Change in Number of Family Gatherings	15
Change in Eating Habits	15
Vacation	13
Christmas Season	12
Minor Violation of the Law	11
Total	

Holmes, T, and Rahe, R: The social readjustment rating scale. *J Psychosom Res,* 11:213, 1967

Physical Stress Symptom Scale

In the space provided, indicate how often each of the following effect happens to you either when you are experiencing stress, or following exposures to a significant stressor. Respond to each item with a number between 0 and 5, using the scale below.

0 = Never　　　　　　　　　　3 = Every few weeks
1 = Once or twice a year　　　4 = Once or more each week
2 = Every few months　　　　 5 = Daily

Cardiovascular Symptoms
____ Heart pounding
____ Heart racing or beating erratically
____ Cold, sweaty hands
____ Headache (throbbing pain)
____ Subtotal

Respiratory Symptoms
____ Rapid, erratic or shallow breathing
____ Shortness of breath
____ Asthma attack
____ Difficulty in speaking because of poor breathing Control
____ Subtotal

Gastrointestinal Symptoms
____ Upset stomach, nausea, or vomiting
____ Constipation
____ Diarrhea
____ Sharp abdominal pains
____ Subtotal

Muscular Symptoms
____ Headaches (steady pain)
____ Back or shoulder pains
____ Muscle tremors or hand shaking
____ Arthritis
____ Subtotal

Skin Symptoms
____ Acne
____ Dandruff
____ Perspiration
____ Excessive dryness of skin or hair
____ Subtotal

Immunity Symptoms
____ Allergy flare-up
____ Catching colds
____ Catching the flu
____ Skin rash
____ Subtotal

Metabolic Symptoms
____ Increased appetite
____ Increased craving for tobacco or sweets
____ Thoughts racing or difficulty sleeping
____ Feelings of crawling anxiety or nervousness
____ Subtotal

____ OVERALL SYMPTOMS TOTAL
(Add all seven subtotals)

From Allen, R: *Progressive neuromuscular relaxation.* Autumn Wind Press. College Park, Md., 1979.

Holmes Inventory

0-149	Mild Stress	30% Chance of Illness
150-299	Moderate Stress	30-80% Chance of Illness
300+	Severe Stress	80% Chance of Illness

Physical Stress Symptom Scale

0-5	No predisposition to disease in that symptom
6-13	Slightly higher risk of disease in that symptom
14+	Likely to experience psychosomatic disease in that symptom

My Final Conclusion, With Best Wishes

One of the goals of this text, and the growth that is expected to accompany working through this text, is to help you grow in self-awareness in order to be less susceptible to professional burnout. Only you can evaluate your current world view, your current level of self-esteem, your current ability to alter harmful perceptions that contribute to negative stress. And only you can change your self-esteem, only you can alter the perceptions about yourself, about the world and about other people to the end that you experience a deep sense of personal confidence and satisfaction in your self and in your work. That is my wish for you. You, your patients, indeed, the world will benefit from the positive energy that you will convey.

You've got a start toward self-awareness and personal growth. Don't stop. Find ways to continue to take regular personal inventory of your self-esteem and your stress levels. Use your journal to stay on top of feelings that would become buried in the overwhelming amount of work you've agreed to do. Make a personal commitment to ongoing growth in all four of your quadrants, and keep a check on the imbalances.

The Signs of Maturation

How will you know when you're succeeding at the maturation process? Someone very wise once offered this description. Life will become more enjoyable, and you will become less worried about making mistakes or not being liked. Relationships will become more important to you than things. You will accept criticism gratefully and graciously, glad for the opportunity to improve. You will not indulge in self-pity, but will begin to see the marvelous opportunities for growth that misfortune and pain often bring. You will not expect special consideration from anyone. You will be aware of your emotions, and you will rarely feel the need to react impulsively in a tense situation. You will meet emergencies with poise; your feelings will not be hurt easily. You will accept responsibility for your own actions without needing to make excuses, readily acknowledging that you are still growing and learning.

You will have grown beyond dualistic, "all or none," "black or white" thinking about the world, and you will be able to tolerate ambiguity. You will recognize that people are doing the best they can, that no one is all bad or all good. You will come to know that true humility is not feeling less important than others, but believing that everyone else is every bit as important as you are.

You will be less impatient with reasonable delay. You will be willing to adjust yourself to others and their needs. You will be gracious losers and will endure defeat without whining or complaining. You will not worry about things you have no control over, and you will learn how to take control of appropriate things with confidence and sensitivity.

You will not need to boast or call attention to yourself. You will feel sincere joy at the success of others, outgrowing both jealousy and envy. And you will be open-minded enough to thoughtfully listen to the thoughts of others.

Above all, you will not tolerate the mistreatment of human beings by those who are careless in their interactions, especially with those who are ill. You will take personal responsibility to help people realize the negative effects of their fragmenting interactions on you and on others, and you will kindly ask them to change their behavior for the good of all concerned. Best of luck to you as you set out to make the world, and yourself, each better than they were when you started.

index